NOOM DIET COO

A Beginner's Guide With 3 Color-Coded Recipes, Meal Plans, And Prep Tips For Beginners And Seniors

Jim Amos

TABLE OF CONTENT

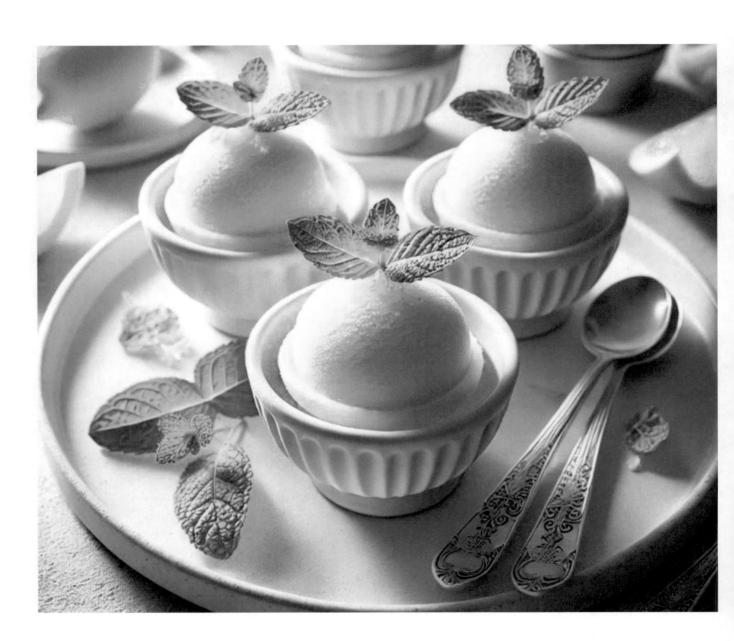

INTRODUCTION

Welcome to the "Noom Diet Cookbook," a culinary journey designed to support your health and wellness goals through the power of mindful eating and balanced nutrition. Whether you're a seasoned Noom user or just beginning your journey, this cookbook is your companion in discovering delicious, satisfying meals that align with the principles of the Noom diet.

The Noom diet is not just about what you eat but how you think about food. It emphasizes the importance of understanding your eating habits, making sustainable lifestyle changes, and fostering a healthy relationship with food. This cookbook embraces those principles by offering recipes that are not only nutritious and wholesome but also enjoyable and easy to prepare.

In this book, you'll find a diverse array of recipes that cater to various tastes and dietary preferences. From hearty breakfasts that kickstart your day to light yet satisfying lunches, vibrant dinners, and delightful snacks, every recipe is crafted with the Noom philosophy in mind. We've focused on using fresh, whole ingredients, vibrant vegetables, lean proteins, and healthy fats to create meals that nourish your body and delight your senses.

The "Noom Diet Cookbook" is more than a collection of recipes; it's a guide to making mindful choices that support your overall well-being. Each recipe is accompanied by tips on portion control, ingredient swaps, and insights into how different foods contribute to your health goals. You'll learn to appreciate the flavors and nutritional benefits of each dish, helping you to build a more intuitive and enjoyable eating experience.

Whether you're cooking for yourself, your family, or friends, this cookbook is designed to inspire you in the kitchen. It's about creating meals that are not only good for your body but also bring joy and satisfaction to your table. With a focus on balance and moderation, the Noom diet encourages you to enjoy a wide variety of foods without feeling deprived.

We invite you to explore the pages of the "Noom Diet Cookbook" with an open mind and a hearty appetite. Let each recipe guide you toward a healthier, happier you, one delicious meal at a time. Happy cooking and bon appétit!

CHAPTER 1

WHAT IS THE NOOM DIET?

The Noom diet is not just another weight loss program; it's a comprehensive lifestyle change that combines psychology, behavioral science, and personalized support to help you achieve your health goals.

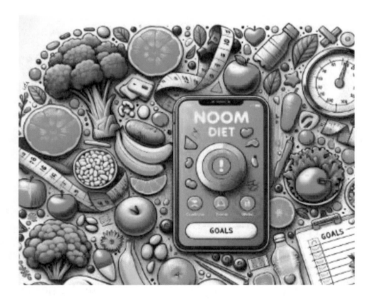

Unlike traditional diets that focus solely on what you eat, Noom emphasizes the importance of why you eat and how you can develop healthier habits for the long term.

Key Principles of the Noom Diet:

- **Behavioral Change:** Noom focuses on helping you understand your eating habits and the psychological triggers behind them. By addressing the root causes of unhealthy eating behaviors, Noom aims to create lasting change.

- **Personalized Approach:** The Noom program tailors its recommendations and support based on your unique needs, preferences, and goals. This personalized approach increases the likelihood of success and helps you stay motivated.

- **Balanced Nutrition:** Rather than categorizing foods as "good" or "bad," Noom encourages a balanced approach to nutrition. It uses a color-coded system (green, yellow, and red) to guide you toward healthier choices without feeling deprived.

- **Support and Accountability:** The Noom app provides access to a community of like-minded individuals, as well as personal coaches who offer guidance, support, and accountability. This social support network is crucial for maintaining motivation and overcoming challenges.

How Noom Works

Understanding how Noom works is essential to fully appreciate its effectiveness and how this cookbook can be a valuable tool in your journey. Here's a closer look at the core components of the Noom program:

The Noom App:

The heart of the Noom program is its user-friendly app, which serves as your personal weight loss coach. The app provides daily lessons, tracking tools, and access to a supportive community. Here's how the app facilitates your journey:

- **Daily Lessons:** Noom offers bite-sized lessons that educate you about nutrition, exercise, and psychological aspects of weight loss. These lessons are designed to be engaging and informative, helping you develop a deeper understanding of healthy living.
- **Tracking Tools:** The app allows you to log your meals, exercise, and weight. By keeping track of your progress, you can identify patterns and make informed decisions about your diet and lifestyle.
- **Color-Coded Food System:** Noom's unique color-coded system categorizes foods into green, yellow, and red groups based on their calorie density and nutritional value. Green foods are the most nutrient-dense and least calorie-dense, yellow foods are moderate, and red foods are the most calorie-dense. This system helps you make healthier choices without feeling restricted.

Psychological Insights:

One of the standout features of Noom is its focus on the psychology of eating. The program helps you recognize and address emotional eating, stress eating, and other psychological triggers that can lead to unhealthy habits. By understanding the "why" behind your eating behaviors, you can develop strategies to manage cravings and make healthier choices.

Personalized Coaching:

Noom provides access to personal coaches who offer tailored advice, support, and accountability. Your coach will work with you to set realistic goals, overcome obstacles, and stay on track. This one-on-one support is invaluable for maintaining motivation and achieving long-term success.

Community Support:

The Noom community is a vibrant, supportive network of individuals who share similar health and weight loss goals. Engaging with the community allows you to share experiences, celebrate successes, and find encouragement during challenging times. This sense of camaraderie is a key factor in maintaining motivation and perseverance

The Psychology of Eating

Understanding the psychology of eating is crucial in the Noom program, which sets it apart from traditional diets. At its core, Noom aims to address the "why" behind your eating habits, recognizing that our relationship with food is deeply rooted in our emotions, environment, and experiences. By exploring these psychological aspects, you can gain insights into your eating behaviors and develop healthier habits.

Emotional Eating:

Emotional eating is a common challenge that many people face. It involves using food as a coping mechanism for emotions such as stress, boredom, sadness, or even happiness. For instance, you might find yourself reaching for a tub of ice cream after a stressful day at work or celebrating a promotion with a lavish meal. While occasional indulgence is normal, relying on food to manage emotions can lead to unhealthy patterns and weight gain.

Noom helps you recognize these emotional triggers by encouraging self-reflection and mindfulness. Through daily lessons and activities, you'll learn to identify when you're eating out of emotion rather than hunger. This awareness is the first step in breaking the cycle of emotional eating. Noom also provides strategies to manage these emotions in healthier ways, such as through exercise, meditation, or talking to a friend.

Cognitive Behavioral Techniques:

Cognitive-behavioral techniques (CBT) are integral to the Noom program. CBT focuses on identifying and changing negative thought patterns that influence behavior. In the context of dieting, these negative thoughts might include self-criticism, all-or-nothing thinking, or catastrophizing about weight gain.

For example, you might think, "I've already ruined my diet by eating that cookie, so I might as well eat the whole bag." Noom teaches you to challenge these thoughts and reframe them in a more positive and realistic light. Instead of spiraling into guilt and overeating, you learn to acknowledge the slip-up and move forward without derailing your progress.

Mindful Eating:

Mindful eating is another key component of the Noom program. It involves paying full attention to the experience of eating, savoring each bite, and listening to your body's hunger and fullness cues. In our fast-paced world, it's easy to eat on autopilot, leading to overconsumption and missed signals of satiety.

Noom encourages practices such as eating without distractions (like TV or smartphones), chewing slowly, and appreciating the flavors and textures of your food. By being more present during meals, you can enjoy your food more and recognize when you're satisfied, preventing overeating.

Calorie Density Explained

Calorie density is a concept central to the Noom diet, playing a pivotal role in how you choose foods and create balanced meals. Understanding calorie density can help you make informed decisions that support weight loss and overall health without feeling deprived.

What is Calorie Density?

Calorie density refers to the number of calories in a given volume or weight of food. Foods with high calorie density have a lot of calories in a small amount of food, while foods with low calorie density have fewer calories in the same volume. This concept is crucial because it allows you to eat satisfying portions of food while managing your calorie intake.

High Calorie Density Foods:

High calorie density foods tend to be rich in fats and sugars, providing a large number of calories in small servings. Examples include:

- **Nuts and seeds:** While nutrient-dense and healthy, nuts and seeds are high in calories.
- **Oils and butter:** Fats are the most calorie-dense macronutrient, so even small amounts can add up quickly.
- **Processed snacks and sweets:** Cookies, chips, and candies are typically high in calories and low in nutritional value.

Low Calorie Density Foods:

Low calorie density foods are typically high in water and fiber, making them filling and nutritious without a high calorie load. Examples include:

- **Fruits and vegetables:** Most fruits and vegetables are low in calories and high in vitamins, minerals, and fiber.
- **Whole grains:** Foods like brown rice, quinoa, and oats are more filling and have fewer calories per serving compared to refined grains.
- **Lean proteins:** Chicken breast, turkey, fish, and legumes are good sources of protein without excessive calories.

Understanding the Noom Color-Coding System

The Noom color-coding system is a simple yet effective way to guide food choices based on their calorie density and nutritional value. Foods are categorized into three groups: green, yellow, and red. This system encourages a balanced diet by promoting nutrient-dense, low-calorie foods while allowing for the occasional indulgence in higher-calorie items. Let's break down each category:

Green Foods: Eat More

Recommended Frequency: Daily

- Percentage of Total Intake: About 30-50% of your daily calories
- Description: These foods are nutrient-dense and lower in calories, so they should make up a significant portion of your diet. They include fruits, vegetables, whole grains, and lean proteins.

Yellow Foods: Eat Moderately

Recommended Frequency: Several times a week

- Percentage of Total Intake: About 30-40% of your daily calories
- Description: These foods have more calories and/or less nutritional value than green foods, so they should be eaten in moderation. They include foods like lean meats, starchy vegetables, and dairy.

Red Foods: Eat Sparingly

Recommended Frequency: Occasionally

- Percentage of Total Intake: About 15-25% of your daily calories
- Description: These foods are higher in calories and often lower in nutritional value, so they should be limited. They include processed foods, sweets, and high-fat meats.

Example of Weekly Plan

Here's an example of how you might structure your weekly eating plan:

Green Foods (Daily)

Aim to include green foods in every meal and snack. For example, start your day with a green smoothie or a bowl of oatmeal with fresh fruits. Include salads, steamed vegetables, and whole grains in your lunch and dinner.

Yellow Foods (Several Times a Week)

Incorporate yellow foods in most meals but in moderate portions. For instance, add lean proteins like chicken or fish to your salads or main dishes, and include starchy vegetables like sweet potatoes a few times a week.

Red Foods (Occasionally)

Save red foods for special occasions or as occasional treats. For example, you might enjoy a dessert or a portion of your favorite high-calorie snack once or twice a week.

CHAPTER 2

BREAKFAST RECIPES (GREEN CODED CODE)

Spinach and Mushroom Scramble

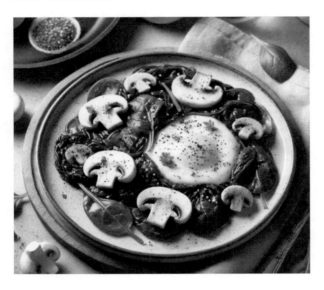

Serves: 1

Cooking Time: 10 minutes

Ingredients and Portions/Measurements:

- Fresh Spinach (Noom diet green color friendly): 1 cup (Packed with vitamins A, C, and K; low in calories)

- White Button Mushrooms (Noom diet green color friendly): 1/2 cup, sliced (Low in calories, high in antioxidants)

- Egg Whites (Substitution for whole eggs to reduce calories and cholesterol): 3 egg whites (High in protein, low in calories)

- Olive Oil Spray (Minimal amount to prevent sticking): Light spray (Healthy fat, use sparingly)

- Garlic Powder (Noom diet green color friendly): 1/4 teaspoon (Adds flavor without calories)

- Black Pepper (Noom diet green color friendly): To taste (Adds flavor without calories)

- Fresh Parsley for garnish (optional) (Noom diet green color friendly): 1 teaspoon, chopped (Adds flavor and nutrients)

Instructions:

- Heat a non-stick skillet over medium heat and lightly spray with olive oil.

- Add the sliced mushrooms to the skillet and sauté for about 3 minutes, or until they begin to soften and release their moisture.

- Add the fresh spinach to the skillet and cook until wilted, about 2 minutes.

- Pour the egg whites into the skillet, and stir gently to combine with the spinach and mushrooms.
- Season with garlic powder and black pepper.
- Continue to cook, stirring occasionally, until the egg whites are fully cooked and set, about 2-3 minutes.
- Transfer the scramble to a plate and garnish with fresh parsley if desired.
- Enjoy your Spinach and Mushroom Scramble warm!

Scientific Note:

Spinach is an excellent ingredient for those on a Noom diet as it is categorized under the green color code, indicating its low-calorie and high-nutrient profile. It is rich in vitamins A, C, and K, which support overall health, including immune function and bone health. The high fiber content in spinach aids in digestion and helps keep you feeling full longer, making it an ideal choice for weight management.

Mushrooms are another green color-coded ingredient in the Noom diet, known for their low-calorie content and high antioxidant levels. They provide essential nutrients such as B vitamins and selenium, which support metabolic function and protect cells from damage.

Egg whites are a lean source of protein, making them perfect for a low-calorie, high-protein breakfast. They help in muscle maintenance and repair without adding extra calories from fat.

This recipe aligns with the Noom diet principles by offering a nutrient-dense meal that is low in calories, helping to support weight loss and overall health.

Nutritional Information (per serving):

- Calories: ~100
- Protein: 12g
- Total Fat: 1g
- Fiber: 2g
- Sodium: Low

Fresh Garden Veggie Scramble

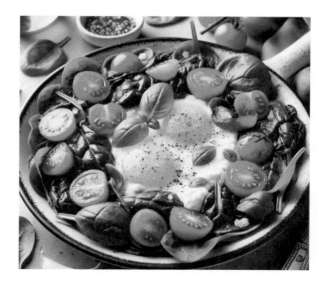

Serves: 1

Cooking Time: 10 minutes

Ingredients and Portions/Measurements:

- Fresh Spinach (Noom diet green color friendly): 1 cup (Packed with vitamins A, C, and K; low in calories)
- Cherry Tomatoes (Noom diet green color friendly): 1/2 cup, halved (Rich in antioxidants, vitamins, and low in calories)
- Egg Whites (Substitution for whole eggs to reduce calories and cholesterol): 3 egg whites (High in protein, low in calories)
- Olive Oil Spray (Minimal amount to prevent sticking): Light spray (Healthy fat, use sparingly)
- Fresh Basil (Noom diet green color friendly): 1 tablespoon, chopped (Adds flavor and nutrients)
- Garlic Powder (Noom diet green color friendly): 1/4 teaspoon (Adds flavor without calories)
- Black Pepper (Noom diet green color friendly): To taste (Adds flavor without calories)

Instructions:

- Heat a non-stick skillet over medium heat and lightly spray with olive oil.
- Add the cherry tomatoes to the skillet and sauté for about 2 minutes, or until they begin to soften.
- Add the fresh spinach to the skillet and cook until wilted, about 2 minutes.
- Pour the egg whites into the skillet, and stir gently to combine with the spinach and tomatoes.
- Season with garlic powder and black pepper.
- Continue to cook, stirring occasionally, until the egg whites are fully cooked and set, about 2-3 minutes.
- Transfer the scramble to a plate and garnish with fresh basil.
- Enjoy your Fresh Garden Veggie Scramble warm!

Scientific Note:

Spinach is a cornerstone of the Noom diet's green-coded foods due to its high nutrient density and low calorie content. It is rich in essential vitamins such as A, C, and K, which contribute to immune function, skin health, and bone strength, respectively. The fiber in spinach aids in digestion and helps maintain satiety, making it an excellent choice for weight management.

Cherry tomatoes, another green-coded food, are packed with antioxidants, particularly lycopene, which has been shown to reduce inflammation and protect against certain chronic diseases. They are also low in calories and high in vitamins A and C, supporting overall health.

Egg whites provide a lean source of protein, which is crucial for muscle maintenance and repair without the added calories and cholesterol found in whole eggs. This makes them an ideal component of a low-calorie, high-protein breakfast that supports weight loss and muscle health.

The combination of these ingredients not only ensures a nutrient-dense meal but also aligns perfectly with the Noom diet principles, promoting weight loss and overall well-being through the consumption of green-coded foods.

Nutritional Information (per serving):

- Calories: ~80
- Protein: 12g
- Total Fat: 1g
- Fiber: 2g
- Sodium: Low

Kale and Apple Breakfast Salad

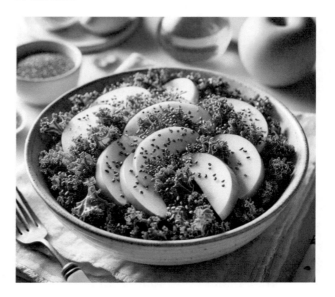

Serves: 1

Cooking Time: 10 minutes

Ingredients and Portions/Measurements:

- Kale (Noom diet green color friendly): 1 cup, chopped (High in vitamins A, C, and K; low in calories)
- Green Apple (Noom diet green color friendly): 1/2 medium apple, thinly sliced (Low in calories, high in fiber and vitamin C)
- Lemon Juice (Noom diet green color friendly): 1 tablespoon (Adds flavor and vitamin C)

- Chia Seeds (Substitution for nuts to keep calories low): 1 teaspoon (High in omega-3 fatty acids and fiber)
- Olive Oil (Minimal amount for dressing): 1/2 teaspoon (Healthy fat, use sparingly)
- Black Pepper (Noom diet green color friendly): To taste (Adds flavor without calories)

Instructions:

- In a large bowl, combine the chopped kale and lemon juice. Massage the kale with your hands for about 2 minutes until it becomes tender.
- Add the thinly sliced green apple to the bowl.
- Drizzle with olive oil and sprinkle with chia seeds.
- Season with black pepper to taste.
- Toss everything together until well combined.
- Enjoy your Kale and Apple Breakfast Salad fresh!

Scientific Note:

Kale is an exceptional green-coded food in the Noom diet due to its low-calorie content and high nutrient density. It is packed with vitamins A, C, and K, which support immune function, skin health, and bone strength, respectively. The fiber in kale aids in digestion and helps

maintain satiety, making it a great choice for weight management.

Green apples are another fantastic green-coded food, offering a crisp, refreshing flavor along with dietary fiber and vitamin C. The fiber helps regulate digestion and prolongs the feeling of fullness, while vitamin C supports the immune system and skin health.

Chia seeds, although used sparingly to keep the calorie count low, provide a significant boost of omega-3 fatty acids and fiber, which are beneficial for heart health and digestion.

This recipe aligns perfectly with the Noom diet principles, providing a nutrient-dense, low-calorie meal that supports weight loss and overall well-being through the consumption of green-coded foods.

Nutritional Information (per serving):

- Calories: ~120
- Protein: 3g
- Total Fat: 5g
- Fiber: 6g
- Sodium: Low

Watermelon Mint Smoothie

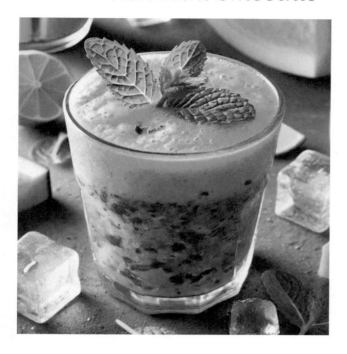

Serves: 1

Cooking Time: 5 minutes

Ingredients and Portions/Measurements:

- Watermelon (Noom diet green color friendly): 1 cup, cubed (Low in calories, high in water content and vitamins A and C)
- Fresh Mint Leaves (Noom diet green color friendly): 5 leaves (Adds refreshing flavor and aids digestion)
- Spinach (Noom diet green color friendly): 1/2 cup (Packed with vitamins A, C, and K; low in calories)
- Ice Cubes (Noom diet green color friendly): 1/2 cup (Adds volume and chill without calories)
- Lime Juice (Noom diet green color friendly): 1 tablespoon (Adds flavor and vitamin C)

Instructions:

- In a blender, combine the cubed watermelon, fresh mint leaves, spinach, ice cubes, and lime juice.
- Blend on high until smooth and well combined.
- Pour the smoothie into a glass.
- Enjoy your Watermelon Mint Smoothie immediately for a refreshing and hydrating breakfast!

Scientific Note:

Watermelon is an excellent choice for the Noom diet's green-coded foods due to its high water content and low calorie count. It provides hydration and is rich in vitamins A and C, which support immune function, skin health, and vision.

Mint leaves not only add a refreshing flavor but also have properties that aid in digestion and provide a sense of calm. They are low in calories and high in nutrients.

Spinach is a nutrient powerhouse, offering a variety of vitamins and minerals with very few calories. It is rich in vitamins A, C, and K, which are essential for immune function, skin health, and bone strength, respectively.

Lime juice adds a zesty flavor to the smoothie while providing a good dose of vitamin C, an antioxidant that helps protect the body from free radicals and supports a healthy immune system.

This smoothie is designed to align with the Noom diet principles by offering a nutrient-dense, low-calorie meal that supports weight loss and overall well-being through the consumption of green-coded foods.

Nutritional Information (per serving):

- Calories: ~60
- Protein: 1g
- Total Fat: 0g
- Fiber: 2g
- Sodium: Low

Cantaloupe and Berry Breakfast Bowl

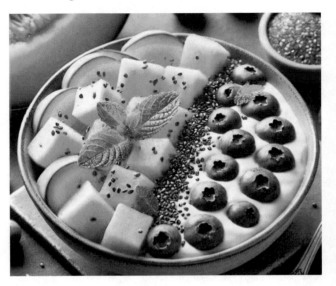

Serves: 1

Cooking Time: 10 minutes

Ingredients and Portions/Measurements:

- Cantaloupe (Noom diet green color friendly): 1 cup, cubed (Low in calories, high in vitamins A and C)
- Blueberries (Noom diet green color friendly): 1/2 cup (Rich in antioxidants and fiber, low in calories)
- Greek Yogurt (Substitution for dairy-free yogurt for lactose intolerance): 1/4 cup (Low in calories and high in protein)
- Chia Seeds (Noom diet green color friendly): 1 teaspoon (High in omega-3 fatty acids and fiber)

- Fresh Mint Leaves (Noom diet green color friendly): 3 leaves, chopped (Adds refreshing flavor and aids digestion)
- Honey (Substitution for a low-calorie sweetener for diabetics): 1 teaspoon (Natural sweetener, use sparingly)

Instructions:

- In a bowl, add the cubed cantaloupe and blueberries.
- Top with Greek yogurt, spreading it evenly over the fruits.
- Sprinkle chia seeds and chopped fresh mint leaves on top.
- Drizzle with honey (or a low-calorie sweetener if preferred).
- Mix gently to combine all ingredients.
- Enjoy your Cantaloupe and Berry Breakfast Bowl immediately!

Scientific Note:

Cantaloupe is an excellent ingredient for the Noom diet due to its low-calorie content and high water percentage, making it a hydrating and refreshing choice. It is rich in vitamins A and C, which are crucial for immune function, skin health, and vision.

Blueberries are another fantastic green-coded food, packed with antioxidants that protect the body from oxidative stress and inflammation. They are also high in fiber, which aids in digestion and promotes a feeling of fullness.

Greek yogurt is a great source of protein, helping to maintain muscle mass and keep you feeling satisfied. It also provides calcium and probiotics, which are beneficial for bone health and digestive health, respectively.

Chia seeds, though used sparingly to keep calories low, provide a significant boost of omega-3 fatty acids and fiber. These nutrients support heart health and digestion.

This recipe aligns with the Noom diet principles by offering a nutrient-dense, low-calorie meal that supports weight loss and overall well-being through the consumption of green-coded foods.

Nutritional Information (per serving):

- Calories: ~150
- Protein: 8g
- Total Fat: 2g
- Fiber: 5g
- Sodium: Low

LUNCH RECIPES (GREEN CODED COLOUR)

Zesty Citrus and Herb Salad

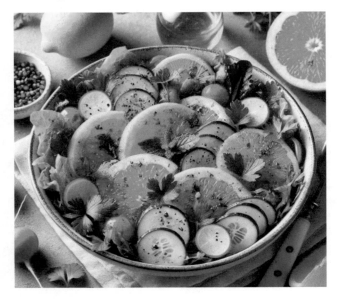

Serves: 1

Cooking Time: 10 minutes

Ingredients and Portions/Measurements:

- Mixed Greens (Noom diet green color friendly): 2 cups (Low in calories, high in vitamins A, C, and K)
- Grapefruit (Noom diet green color friendly): 1/2 medium grapefruit, segmented (Low in calories, high in vitamin C and fiber)
- Cucumber (Noom diet green color friendly): 1/2 cup, sliced (Low in calories, high in water content and vitamins)
- Radishes (Noom diet green color friendly): 1/4 cup, thinly sliced (Low in calories, high in vitamin C and fiber)
- Fresh Mint (Noom diet green color friendly): 1 tablespoon, chopped (Adds refreshing flavor and aids digestion)
- Fresh Parsley (Noom diet green color friendly): 1 tablespoon, chopped (Rich in vitamins A, C, and K)
- Olive Oil (Minimal amount for dressing): 1 teaspoon (Healthy fat, use sparingly)
- Fresh Lemon Juice (Noom diet green color friendly): 1 tablespoon (Adds flavor and vitamin C)
- Black Pepper (Noom diet green color friendly): To taste (Adds flavor without calories)

Instructions:

- In a large bowl, combine the mixed greens, segmented grapefruit, sliced cucumber, and sliced radishes.
- Add the chopped fresh mint and parsley to the bowl.
- Drizzle with olive oil and fresh lemon juice.
- Season with black pepper to taste.

- Toss everything together until well combined.
- Enjoy your Zesty Citrus and Herb Salad immediately for a refreshing and nutritious lunch!

Scientific Note:

Mixed greens are a cornerstone of the Noom diet's green color-coded foods due to their low-calorie content and high nutrient density. They provide essential vitamins such as A, C, and K, which support immune function, skin health, and bone strength, respectively. The fiber in mixed greens aids in digestion and helps maintain satiety, making them an excellent choice for weight management.

Grapefruit is a hydrating, low-calorie fruit rich in vitamin C and fiber. Vitamin C acts as an antioxidant, protecting the body from free radicals and boosting the immune system. The fiber content helps regulate digestion and prolongs the feeling of fullness, making grapefruit an ideal fruit for weight loss.

This recipe aligns with the Noom diet principles by offering a nutrient-dense, low-calorie meal that supports weight loss and overall well-being through the consumption of green-coded foods.

Nutritional Information (per serving):

- Calories: ~120
- Protein: 2g
- Total Fat: 4g
- Fiber: 6g
- Sodium: Low

Zucchini Noodles with Lemon Herb Dressing

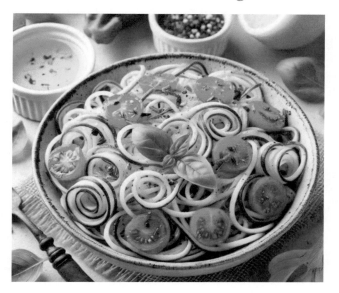

Serves: 1

Cooking Time: 10 minutes

Ingredients and Portions/Measurements:

- Zucchini (Noom diet green color friendly): 1 medium zucchini, spiralized (Low in calories, high in vitamins and fiber)
- Cherry Tomatoes (Noom diet green color friendly): 1/2 cup, halved (Rich in vitamins A and C, low in calories)
- Fresh Basil (Noom diet green color friendly): 1 tablespoon, chopped (Adds flavor and nutrients)

- Fresh Lemon Juice (Noom diet green color friendly): 1 tablespoon (Adds flavor and vitamin C)
- Olive Oil (Minimal amount for dressing): 1 teaspoon (Healthy fat, use sparingly)
- Garlic Powder (Noom diet green color friendly): 1/4 teaspoon (Adds flavor without calories)
- Black Pepper (Noom diet green color friendly): To taste (Adds flavor without calories)

Instructions:

- Spiralize the zucchini to create zucchini noodles. If you don't have a spiralizer, you can use a vegetable peeler to create thin strips.
- Place the zucchini noodles in a large bowl.
- Add the halved cherry tomatoes and chopped fresh basil to the bowl.
- In a small bowl, whisk together the fresh lemon juice, olive oil, garlic powder, and black pepper to make the dressing.
- Pour the dressing over the zucchini noodles and toss gently to combine.
- Serve immediately and enjoy your Zucchini Noodles with Lemon Herb Dressing!

Scientific Note:

Zucchini is an excellent choice for a low-calorie, nutrient-dense meal. It is high in vitamins A and C, which support immune function and skin health, and it contains fiber that aids in digestion and helps maintain a feeling of fullness.

Cherry tomatoes are another green-coded food in the Noom diet, packed with antioxidants and vitamins A and C. They are low in calories and add a sweet, tangy flavor to the dish.

Fresh basil not only enhances the flavor of the meal but also provides essential vitamins and minerals. It is rich in vitamin K, which is important for bone health, and it contains antioxidants that support overall health.

This recipe aligns with the Noom diet principles, offering a nutrient-dense, low-calorie meal that supports weight loss and overall well-being through the consumption of green-coded foods.

Nutritional Information (per serving):

- Calories: ~70
- Protein: 2g
- Total Fat: 3g
- Fiber: 2g
- Sodium: Low

Asian-Inspired Cabbage Wraps

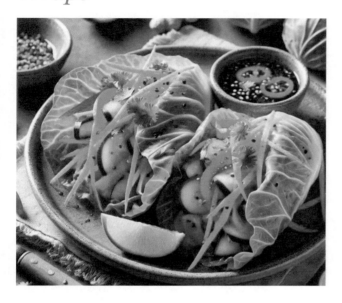

Serves: 1

Cooking Time: 10 minutes

Ingredients and Portions/Measurements:

- Green Cabbage Leaves (Noom diet green color friendly): 2 large leaves (Low in calories, high in fiber and vitamins)
- Carrot (Noom diet green color friendly): 1/4 cup, julienned (High in beta-carotene and fiber, low in calories)
- Red Bell Pepper (Noom diet green color friendly): 1/4 cup, thinly sliced (Rich in vitamins A and C, low in calories)
- Cucumber (Noom diet green color friendly): 1/4 cup, thinly sliced (Low in calories, high in water content and vitamins)
- Fresh Cilantro (Noom diet green color friendly): 1 tablespoon, chopped (Adds flavor and nutrients)
- Fresh Lime Juice (Noom diet green color friendly): 1 tablespoon (Adds flavor and vitamin C)
- Soy Sauce (Low-sodium for health benefits): 1 teaspoon (Adds flavor)
- Fresh Ginger (Noom diet green color friendly): 1/2 teaspoon, grated (Adds flavor and has anti-inflammatory properties)
- Black Pepper (Noom diet green color friendly): To taste (Adds flavor without calories)

Instructions:

- Lay the cabbage leaves flat and spread them out to use as wraps.
- In a bowl, combine the julienned carrot, sliced red bell pepper, sliced cucumber, and chopped fresh cilantro.
- In a small bowl, mix the fresh lime juice, soy sauce, grated fresh ginger, and black pepper to make the dressing.
- Drizzle the dressing over the vegetable mixture and toss to combine.

- Place the vegetable mixture in the center of each cabbage leaf.
- Fold the sides of the cabbage leaves over the filling and roll them up to form wraps.
- Enjoy your Asian-Inspired Cabbage Wraps immediately for a light and refreshing lunch!

Scientific Note:

Cabbage is an excellent low-calorie vegetable that provides a good amount of fiber, vitamins C and K, and various antioxidants. It is perfect for weight management due to its high nutrient density and low calorie count.

Carrots are rich in beta-carotene, fiber, and antioxidants, supporting overall health and vision. Their natural sweetness adds flavor and texture to the wraps.

Red bell peppers are packed with vitamins A and C, which are crucial for immune function and skin health. They are low in calories and add a crisp texture to the dish.

This recipe aligns with the Noom diet principles by offering a nutrient-dense, low-calorie meal that supports weight loss and overall well-being through the consumption of green-coded foods.

Nutritional Information (per serving):

- Calories: ~60
- Protein: 2g
- Total Fat: 0.5g
- Fiber: 4g
- Sodium: Low

Tangy Radish and Herb Salad

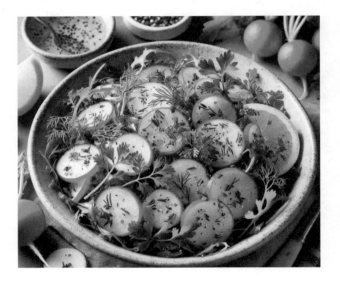

Serves: 1

Cooking Time: 10 minutes

Ingredients and Portions/Measurements:

- Radishes (Noom diet green color friendly): 1 cup, thinly sliced (Low in calories, high in fiber and vitamin C)
- Arugula (Noom diet green color friendly): 1 cup (Low in calories, high in vitamins A and K)

- Fresh Parsley (Noom diet green color friendly): 2 tablespoons, chopped (Adds flavor and nutrients)
- Fresh Dill (Noom diet green color friendly): 1 tablespoon, chopped (Adds flavor and nutrients)
- Lemon Juice (Noom diet green color friendly): 1 tablespoon (Adds flavor and vitamin C)
- Olive Oil (Minimal amount for dressing): 1 teaspoon (Healthy fat, use sparingly)
- Black Pepper (Noom diet green color friendly): To taste (Adds flavor without calories)

Instructions:

- In a large bowl, combine the thinly sliced radishes, arugula, chopped fresh parsley, and chopped fresh dill.
- In a small bowl, whisk together the lemon juice, olive oil, and black pepper to make the dressing.
- Pour the dressing over the salad and toss gently to combine.
- Serve immediately and enjoy your Tangy Radish and Herb Salad!

Scientific Note:

Radishes are a low-calorie, nutrient-dense vegetable that provides a good amount of vitamin C, fiber, and antioxidants. They help promote digestion and support immune function, making them an excellent choice for weight management.

Arugula is another green-coded food in the Noom diet, known for its low calorie content and high levels of vitamins A and K. These vitamins support vision, immune function, and bone health, respectively. Arugula also contains antioxidants that help protect cells from damage.

This recipe aligns with the Noom diet principles by offering a nutrient-dense, low-calorie meal that supports weight loss and overall well-being through the consumption of green-coded foods.

Nutritional Information (per serving):

- Calories: ~50
- Protein: 2g
- Total Fat: 2g
- Fiber: 3g
- Sodium: Low

Mango and Cucumber Summer Roll

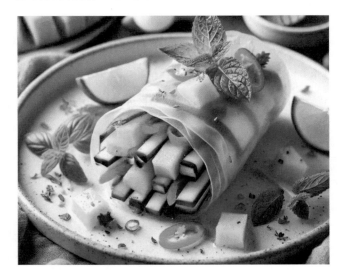

Serves: 1

Cooking Time: 10 minutes

Ingredients and Portions/Measurements:

- Rice Paper Wraps (Noom diet green color friendly): 2 sheets (Low in calories, gluten-free)
- Mango (Noom diet green color friendly): 1/4 cup, thinly sliced (Low in calories, high in vitamins A and C)
- Cucumber (Noom diet green color friendly): 1/4 cup, julienned (Low in calories, high in water content and vitamins)
- Red Bell Pepper (Noom diet green color friendly): 1/4 cup, thinly sliced (Rich in vitamins A and C, low in calories)
- Fresh Mint Leaves (Noom diet green color friendly): 1 tablespoon, chopped (Adds refreshing flavor and aids digestion)
- Fresh Basil Leaves (Noom diet green color friendly): 1 tablespoon, chopped (Adds flavor and nutrients)
- Fresh Lime Juice (Noom diet green color friendly): 1 tablespoon (Adds flavor and vitamin C)
- Soy Sauce (Low-sodium for health benefits): 1 teaspoon (Adds flavor)
- Water (For softening rice paper wraps)

Instructions:

- Fill a large shallow dish with warm water. Submerge one rice paper wrap in the water for about 15-20 seconds, or until it becomes pliable. Remove and place on a clean surface.
- Arrange half of the mango slices, cucumber, red bell pepper, mint leaves, and basil leaves in the center of the softened rice paper wrap.
- Drizzle with half of the fresh lime juice and a tiny bit of soy sauce.
- Fold the sides of the rice paper wrap over the filling, then roll tightly from the bottom to the top to enclose the filling completely.

- Repeat with the second rice paper wrap and remaining ingredients.
- Serve immediately and enjoy your Mango and Cucumber Summer Roll!

Scientific Note:

Rice paper wraps are a low-calorie, gluten-free option perfect for making light and refreshing rolls. They provide a versatile base for a variety of nutrient-dense fillings.

Mango is a delicious tropical fruit that is low in calories and rich in vitamins A and C. These vitamins are crucial for immune function, skin health, and vision. Mango also contains dietary fiber, which aids digestion and helps maintain a feeling of fullness.

This recipe aligns with the Noom diet principles by offering a nutrient-dense, low-calorie meal that supports weight loss and overall well-being through the consumption of green-coded foods.

Nutritional Information (per serving):

- Calories: ~80
- Protein: 1g
- Total Fat: 0.5g
- Fiber: 2g
- Sodium: Low

DINNER RECIPE

(GREEN CODED COLOR)

Cauliflower Rice Stir-Fry

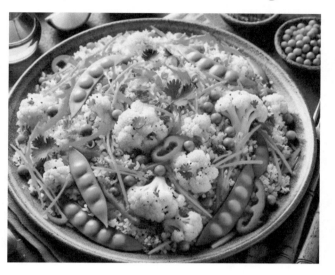

serves: 1

Cooking Time: 15 minutes

Ingredients and Portions/Measurements:

- Cauliflower (Noom diet green color friendly): 1 cup, riced (Low in calories, high in vitamins and fiber)
- Snap Peas (Noom diet green color friendly): 1/2 cup, trimmed (Low in calories, high in vitamins and fiber)
- Carrot (Noom diet green color friendly): 1/4 cup, julienned (High in beta-carotene and fiber, low in calories)

- Red Bell Pepper (Noom diet green color friendly): 1/4 cup, thinly sliced (Rich in vitamins A and C, low in calories)
- Green Onions (Noom diet green color friendly): 1 tablespoon, chopped (Adds flavor and nutrients)
- Fresh Ginger (Noom diet green color friendly): 1 teaspoon, grated (Adds flavor and has anti-inflammatory properties)
- Garlic (Noom diet green color friendly): 1 clove, minced (Adds flavor and has health benefits)
- Soy Sauce (Low-sodium for health benefits): 1 teaspoon (Adds flavor)
- Olive Oil Spray (Minimal amount to prevent sticking): Light spray (Healthy fat, use sparingly)
- Fresh Cilantro (Noom diet green color friendly): 1 tablespoon, chopped (Adds flavor and nutrients)
- Lime Wedge (Noom diet green color friendly): 1 wedge (Adds flavor and vitamin C)

Instructions:

- Heat a non-stick skillet over medium heat and lightly spray with olive oil.
- Add the minced garlic and grated ginger to the skillet and sauté for about 1 minute, or until fragrant.
- Add the riced cauliflower, snap peas, julienned carrot, and sliced red bell pepper to the skillet. Stir-fry for about 5-7 minutes, or until the vegetables are tender-crisp.
- Stir in the chopped green onions and soy sauce, cooking for another 1-2 minutes until everything is well combined and heated through.
- Remove from heat and sprinkle with fresh cilantro.
- Serve with a lime wedge on the side to squeeze over the stir-fry for an extra burst of flavor.
- Enjoy your Cauliflower Rice Stir-Fry immediately!

Scientific Note:

Cauliflower is a fantastic low-calorie substitute for rice, making it perfect for a light dinner. It is high in fiber, which aids in digestion and helps maintain a feeling of fullness. Cauliflower is also rich in vitamins C and K, supporting immune function and bone health.

Snap peas and carrots are nutrient-dense vegetables that provide vitamins A and C, fiber, and antioxidants. These nutrients help protect the body from oxidative stress and support overall health.

Red bell peppers add vibrant color and are packed with vitamins A and C, crucial for immune function and skin health. They are low in calories and high in antioxidants.

Garlic and ginger not only add a burst of flavor

This recipe aligns with the Noom diet principles by offering a nutrient-dense, low-calorie meal that supports weight loss and overall well-being through the consumption of green-coded foods.

Nutritional Information (per serving):

- Calories: ~100
- Protein: 3g
- Total Fat: 1g
- Fiber: 5g
- Sodium: Low

Spinach and Mushroom Stuffed Portobello

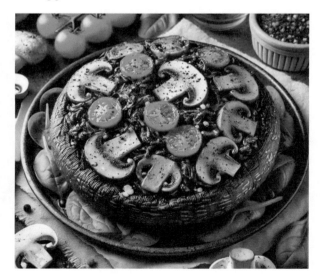

Serves: 1

Cooking Time: 20 minutes

Ingredients and Portions/Measurements:

- Portobello Mushroom Cap (Noom diet green color friendly): 1 large cap, cleaned and stem removed (Low in calories, rich in antioxidants and fiber)
- Spinach (Noom diet green color friendly): 1 cup, chopped (Packed with vitamins A, C, and K; low in calories)
- Button Mushrooms (Noom diet green color friendly): 1/4 cup, diced (Low in calories, high in antioxidants)
- Cherry Tomatoes (Noom diet green color friendly): 1/4 cup, halved (Rich in vitamins A and C, low in calories)
- Garlic (Noom diet green color friendly): 1 clove, minced (Adds flavor and has health benefits)
- Olive Oil Spray (Minimal amount to prevent sticking): Light spray (Healthy fat, use sparingly)
- Black Pepper (Noom diet green color friendly): To taste (Adds flavor without calories)
- Fresh Basil (Noom diet green color friendly): 1 tablespoon, chopped (Adds flavor and nutrients)
- Balsamic Vinegar (Optional): 1 teaspoon (Adds flavor and low in calories)

Instructions:

- Preheat the oven to 375°F (190°C).
- Lightly spray a baking sheet with olive oil.
- Place the portobello mushroom cap on the baking sheet, gill side up.
- In a non-stick skillet over medium heat, lightly spray with olive oil. Add the minced garlic and sauté for about 1 minute until fragrant.
- Add the diced button mushrooms and halved cherry tomatoes to the skillet. Cook for about 3-4 minutes until softened.
- Add the chopped spinach to the skillet and cook until wilted, about 2 minutes.
- Season the mixture with black pepper and remove from heat.
- Spoon the spinach and mushroom mixture into the portobello mushroom cap.
- Bake in the preheated oven for 10-12 minutes, or until the portobello is tender.
- Remove from the oven and sprinkle with fresh basil.
- Drizzle with balsamic vinegar if desired.
- Serve immediately and enjoy your Spinach and Mushroom Stuffed Portobello!

Scientific Note:

Portobello mushrooms are an excellent low-calorie option that provides a substantial and satisfying base for a variety of fillings. They are rich in antioxidants and fiber, supporting overall health and digestion.

Spinach is a nutrient powerhouse, offering a variety of vitamins and minerals with very few calories. It is rich in vitamins A, C, and K, which support immune function, skin health, and bone strength, respectively.

Button mushrooms are another low-calorie, nutrient-dense food that adds volume and texture to meals without adding many calories. They are high in antioxidants and vitamins, supporting overall health.

This recipe aligns with the Noom diet principles by offering a nutrient-dense, low-calorie meal that supports weight loss and overall well-being through the consumption of green-coded foods.

Nutritional Information (per serving):

- Calories: ~90
- Protein: 4g
- Total Fat: 1.5g
- Fiber: 3g
- Sodium: Low

Eggplant and Tomato Bake

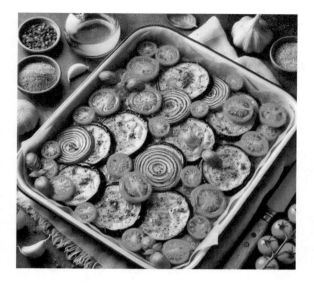

Serves: 1

Cooking Time: 25 minutes

Ingredients and Portions/Measurements:

- Eggplant (Noom diet green color friendly): 1 small, sliced into rounds (Low in calories, high in fiber and antioxidants)
- Cherry Tomatoes (Noom diet green color friendly): 1/2 cup, halved (Rich in vitamins A and C, low in calories)
- Red Onion (Noom diet green color friendly): 1/4 cup, thinly sliced (Adds flavor and nutrients)
- Garlic (Noom diet green color friendly): 1 clove, minced (Adds flavor and has health benefits)

- Olive Oil Spray (Minimal amount to prevent sticking): Light spray (Healthy fat, use sparingly)
- Fresh Basil (Noom diet green color friendly): 1 tablespoon, chopped (Adds flavor and nutrients)
- Black Pepper (Noom diet green color friendly): To taste (Adds flavor without calories)
- Balsamic Vinegar (Optional): 1 teaspoon (Adds flavor and low in calories)

Instructions:

- Preheat the oven to 400°F (200°C).
- Lightly spray a baking dish with olive oil.
- Arrange the eggplant slices in a single layer in the baking dish.
- Top with the halved cherry tomatoes and thinly sliced red onion.
- Sprinkle the minced garlic evenly over the vegetables.
- Lightly spray the top with olive oil and season with black pepper.
- Bake in the preheated oven for 20 minutes, or until the eggplant is tender and the tomatoes are roasted.
- Remove from the oven and sprinkle with fresh basil.
- Drizzle with balsamic vinegar if desired.

- Serve immediately and enjoy your Eggplant and Tomato Bake!

Scientific Note:

Eggplant is a nutrient-dense, low-calorie vegetable rich in fiber, which aids in digestion and helps maintain a feeling of fullness. It also contains antioxidants that protect the body from oxidative stress and support overall health.

Cherry tomatoes are packed with vitamins A and C, essential for immune function, skin health, and vision. They are low in calories and high in antioxidants, making them a perfect addition to a weight loss diet.

Red onions add a flavorful kick and are rich in antioxidants, vitamins, and minerals. They support heart health and have anti-inflammatory properties.

This recipe aligns with the Noom diet principles by offering a nutrient-dense, low-calorie meal that supports weight loss and overall well-being through the consumption of green-coded foods.

Nutritional Information (per serving):

- Calories: ˜80
- Protein: 2g
- Total Fat: 1g
- Fiber: 4g
- Sodium: Low

Cabbage and Carrot Stir-Fry

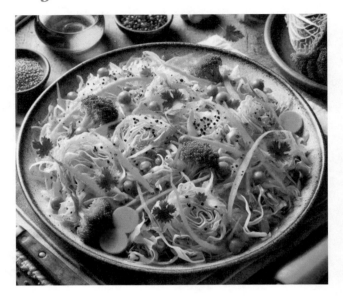

Serves: 1

Cooking Time: 15 minutes

Ingredients and Portions/Measurements:

- Green Cabbage (Noom diet green color friendly): 1 cup, thinly sliced (Low in calories, high in fiber and vitamins)
- Carrot (Noom diet green color friendly): 1/4 cup, julienned (High in beta-carotene and fiber, low in calories)
- Green Onion (Noom diet green color friendly): 1 tablespoon, chopped (Adds flavor and nutrients)
- Fresh Ginger (Noom diet green color friendly): 1 teaspoon, grated (Adds flavor and has anti-inflammatory properties)

- Garlic (Noom diet green color friendly): 1 clove, minced (Adds flavor and has health benefits)
- Soy Sauce (Low-sodium for health benefits): 1 teaspoon (Adds flavor)
- Olive Oil Spray (Minimal amount to prevent sticking): Light spray (Healthy fat, use sparingly)
- Black Pepper (Noom diet green color friendly): To taste (Adds flavor without calories)
- Fresh Cilantro (Noom diet green color friendly): 1 tablespoon, chopped (Adds flavor and nutrients)

Instructions:

- Heat a non-stick skillet over medium heat and lightly spray with olive oil.
- Add the minced garlic and grated ginger to the skillet and sauté for about 1 minute until fragrant.
- Add the thinly sliced cabbage and julienned carrot to the skillet. Stir-fry for about 5-7 minutes, or until the vegetables are tender-crisp.
- Add the chopped green onion and low-sodium soy sauce. Cook for another 1-2 minutes until everything is well combined and heated through.
- Season with black pepper to taste.
- Remove from heat and sprinkle with fresh cilantro.
- Serve immediately and enjoy your Cabbage and Carrot Stir-Fry!

Scientific Note:

Green cabbage is an excellent low-calorie vegetable that is high in fiber, which aids in digestion and helps maintain a feeling of fullness. It is also rich in vitamins C and K, which support immune function and bone health.

Carrots are packed with beta-carotene, fiber, and antioxidants. Beta-carotene is converted into vitamin A in the body, which is crucial for vision and immune function. Carrots' fiber content also aids in digestion and promotes satiety.

Green onions add a mild flavor and are rich in vitamins A and K, which support vision and bone health.

This recipe aligns with the Noom diet principles by offering a nutrient-dense, low-calorie meal that supports weight loss and overall well-being through the consumption of green-coded foods.

Nutritional Information (per serving):

- Calories: ~70
- Protein: 2g
- Total Fat: 1g
- Fiber: 4g

- Sodium: Low

Lemon Herb Zoodle Salad

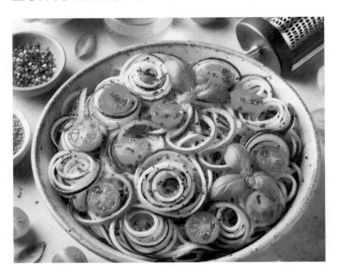

Serves: 1

Cooking Time: 15 minutes

Ingredients and Portions/Measurements:

- Zucchini (Noom diet green color friendly): 1 medium, spiralized into zoodles (Low in calories, high in vitamins and fiber)
- Cherry Tomatoes (Noom diet green color friendly): 1/2 cup, halved (Rich in vitamins A and C, low in calories)
- Red Onion (Noom diet green color friendly): 1/4 cup, thinly sliced (Adds flavor and nutrients)
- Fresh Basil (Noom diet green color friendly): 2 tablespoons, chopped (Adds flavor and nutrients)
- Fresh Parsley (Noom diet green color friendly): 1 tablespoon, chopped (Adds flavor and nutrients)
- Fresh Lemon Juice (Noom diet green color friendly): 1 tablespoon (Adds flavor and vitamin C)
- Olive Oil (Minimal amount for dressing): 1 teaspoon (Healthy fat, use sparingly)
- Garlic Powder (Noom diet green color friendly): 1/4 teaspoon (Adds flavor without calories)

Black Pepper (Noom diet green color friendly): To taste (Adds flavor without calories)

Instructions:

- Spiralize the zucchini into zoodles using a spiralizer or julienne peeler.
- In a large bowl, combine the zucchini zoodles, halved cherry tomatoes, and thinly sliced red onion.
- In a small bowl, whisk together the fresh lemon juice, olive oil, garlic powder, and black pepper to make the dressing.
- Pour the dressing over the zoodle salad and toss gently to combine.
- Sprinkle the chopped fresh basil and parsley over the top.
- Serve immediately and enjoy your Lemon Herb Zoodle Salad!

Scientific Note:

Zucchini is an excellent low-calorie vegetable that is high in vitamins and minerals, making it perfect for a light and healthy meal. It is rich in vitamins A and C, which support immune function and skin health, and fiber, which aids in digestion and promotes a feeling of fullness.

Cherry tomatoes are another nutrient-dense, low-calorie food. They are packed with vitamins A and C, antioxidants that help protect the body from oxidative stress and support overall health.

Red onions add a flavorful kick and are rich in antioxidants, vitamins, and minerals. They support heart health and have anti-inflammatory properties.

This recipe aligns with the Noom diet principles by offering a nutrient-dense, low-calorie meal that supports weight loss and overall well-being through the consumption of green-coded foods.

Nutritional Information (per serving):

- Calories: ~60
- Protein: 2g
- Total Fat: 1g
- Fiber: 3g
- Sodium: Low

Banana Almond Overnight Oats

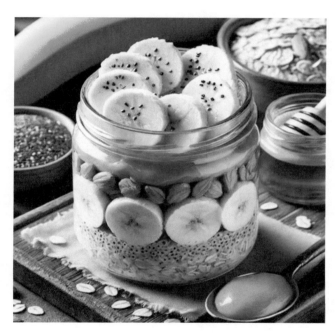

Serves: 1

Cooking Time: 5 minutes (plus overnight refrigeration)

Ingredients and Portions/Measurements:

- Rolled Oats (Noom diet yellow food friendly): 1/2 cup (Rich in fiber and whole grains, helps maintain satiety)
- Almond Milk (Noom diet yellow food friendly): 1/2 cup (Low in calories, high in vitamins and minerals)
- Banana (Noom diet yellow food friendly): 1/2 medium, sliced (Provides natural sweetness, rich in potassium and fiber)
- Almond Butter (Noom diet yellow food friendly): 1 tablespoon (Adds healthy fats and protein)
- Chia Seeds (Noom diet yellow food friendly): 1 teaspoon (High in omega-3 fatty acids and fiber)
- Honey (Noom diet yellow food friendly): 1 teaspoon (Natural sweetener, use sparingly)

Instructions:

- In a mason jar or small bowl, combine the rolled oats, almond milk, and chia seeds.
- Stir well to ensure the chia seeds are evenly distributed.
- Add the sliced banana on top of the oat mixture.
- Drizzle the almond butter over the banana slices.
- Add a teaspoon of honey for natural sweetness.
- Cover the jar or bowl and refrigerate overnight.
- In the morning, stir the mixture and enjoy your Banana Almond Overnight Oats cold.

Scientific Note:

Rolled oats are an excellent source of complex carbohydrates and fiber, particularly beta-glucan, which can help lower cholesterol levels and stabilize blood sugar. Oats provide a slow release of energy, keeping you full longer and aiding in weight management.

Almond milk is a nutritious alternative to dairy milk, providing vitamins E and D, as well as calcium. It is low in calories and suitable for those with lactose intolerance or dairy allergies.

Bananas add natural sweetness and are rich in potassium, an essential mineral for heart health and muscle function. Their fiber content helps promote digestive health and provides a feeling of fullness.

This recipe aligns with the Noom diet principles by offering a balanced, nutrient-dense meal that supports weight loss and overall well-being through the consumption of yellow-coded foods.

Nutritional Information (per serving):

- Calories: ~300
- Protein: 8g

- Total Fat: 10g
- Fiber: 7g
- Sodium: Low

Sweet Potato and Spinach Breakfast Hash

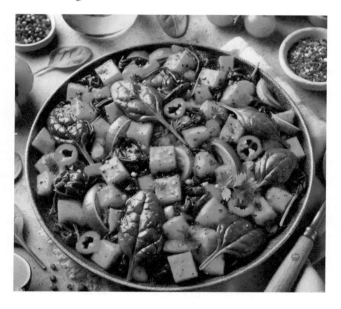

Serves: 1

Cooking Time: 20 minutes

Ingredients and Portions/Measurements:

- Sweet Potato (Noom diet yellow food friendly): 1 small, diced (Rich in vitamins A and C, provides fiber and complex carbohydrates)
- Spinach (Noom diet yellow food friendly): 1 cup, chopped (Rich in vitamins A, C, and K; low in calories)
- Red Bell Pepper (Noom diet yellow food friendly): 1/4 cup, diced (Rich in vitamins A and C, low in calories)
- Olive Oil (Minimal amount for cooking): 1 teaspoon (Healthy fat, use sparingly)
- Red Onion (Noom diet yellow food friendly): 1/4 cup, diced (Adds flavor and nutrients)
- Garlic (Noom diet yellow food friendly): 1 clove, minced (Adds flavor and has health benefits)
- Black Pepper (Noom diet yellow food friendly): To taste (Adds flavor without calories)
- Fresh Parsley (Noom diet yellow food friendly): 1 tablespoon, chopped (Adds flavor and nutrients)

Instructions:

- Heat a non-stick skillet over medium heat and add the olive oil.
- Add the diced sweet potato to the skillet and cook for about 10 minutes, stirring occasionally, until the sweet potato is tender and slightly crispy.
- Add the diced red onion, red bell pepper, and minced garlic to the skillet. Cook for another 5 minutes, or until the vegetables are softened.

- Add the chopped spinach to the skillet and cook until wilted, about 2 minutes.
- Season with black pepper to taste.
- Remove from heat and sprinkle with fresh parsley.
- Serve immediately and enjoy your Sweet Potato and Spinach Breakfast Hash!

Scientific Note:

Sweet potatoes are an excellent source of complex carbohydrates, providing a slow release of energy that helps maintain blood sugar levels and keeps you feeling full longer. They are rich in vitamins A and C, which support immune function, skin health, and vision.

Spinach is packed with vitamins A, C, and K, which are crucial for immune function, skin health, and bone strength. Its high fiber content aids in digestion and promotes satiety.

Red bell peppers add vibrant color and are loaded with vitamins A and C, antioxidants that help protect the body from oxidative stress and support overall health. They are low in calories and high in fiber.

This recipe aligns with the Noom diet principles by offering a nutrient-dense, moderate-calorie meal that supports weight loss and overall well-being through the consumption of yellow-coded foods.

Nutritional Information (per serving):

- Calories: ~250

- Protein: 4g
- Total Fat: 5g
- Fiber: 6g
- Sodium: Low

Greek Yogurt Parfait with Granola and Berries

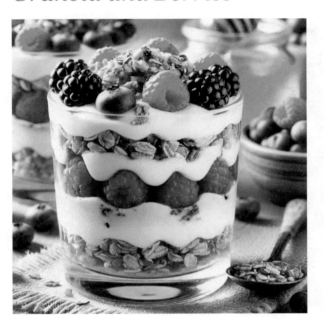

Serves: 1

Cooking Time: 5 minutes

Ingredients and Portions/Measurements:

- Greek Yogurt (Noom diet yellow food friendly): 1/2 cup (High in protein, low in fat)
- Granola (Noom diet yellow food friendly): 1/4 cup (Provides fiber and healthy carbs)
- Fresh Mixed Berries (Noom diet yellow food friendly): 1/2 cup (Rich in

antioxidants, vitamins, and low in calories)

- Honey (Noom diet yellow food friendly): 1 teaspoon (Natural sweetener, use sparingly)
- Chia Seeds (Optional, tolerated by few): 1 teaspoon (Substitute with flax seeds for a different texture and nutrients)

Instructions:

- In a glass or bowl, layer half of the Greek yogurt at the bottom.
- Add a layer of granola over the yogurt.
- Add a layer of fresh mixed berries on top of the granola.
- Repeat the layers with the remaining Greek yogurt, granola, and berries.
- Drizzle honey over the top layer of berries.
- Sprinkle chia seeds or flax seeds on top if desired.
- Serve immediately and enjoy your Greek Yogurt Parfait with Granola and Berries!

Scientific Note:

Greek yogurt is an excellent source of protein, which helps keep you full and supports muscle maintenance. It is low in fat and provides calcium and probiotics, which are beneficial for bone and gut health.

Granola, when chosen carefully to avoid added sugars, provides a good source of fiber and healthy carbohydrates. Fiber aids in digestion and helps maintain satiety, which is beneficial for weight management.

Fresh mixed berries are packed with antioxidants, which help protect the body from oxidative stress and inflammation. They are low in calories and high in vitamins, particularly vitamins C and K, supporting immune function and skin health.

This recipe aligns with the Noom diet principles by offering a nutrient-dense, moderate-calorie meal that supports weight loss and overall well-being through the consumption of yellow-coded foods.

Nutritional Information (per serving):

- Calories: ~300
- Protein: 15g
- Total Fat: 8g
- Fiber: 7g
- Sodium: Low

Apple Cinnamon Oatmeal

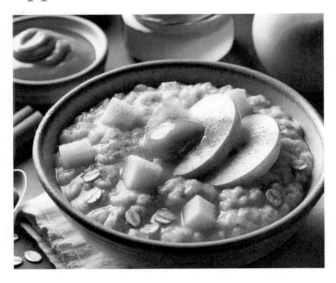

Serves: 1

Cooking Time: 10 minutes

Ingredients and Portions/Measurements:

- Rolled Oats (Noom diet yellow food friendly): 1/2 cup (Rich in fiber and whole grains, helps maintain satiety)
- Water: 1 cup (For cooking oats)
- Apple (Noom diet yellow food friendly): 1/2 medium, diced (Provides natural sweetness, rich in fiber and vitamins)
- Cinnamon (Noom diet yellow food friendly): 1/2 teaspoon (Adds flavor and has anti-inflammatory properties)
- Almond Butter (Noom diet yellow food friendly): 1 tablespoon (Adds healthy fats and protein)

- Honey (Noom diet yellow food friendly): 1 teaspoon (Natural sweetener, use sparingly)

Instructions:

- In a small saucepan, bring the water to a boil.
- Add the rolled oats and reduce the heat to a simmer. Cook for about 5 minutes, stirring occasionally, until the oats are soft and the water is absorbed.
- Stir in the diced apple and cinnamon, cooking for another 2-3 minutes until the apple is slightly softened.
- Remove from heat and transfer the oatmeal to a bowl.
- Drizzle the almond butter and honey over the top.
- Serve immediately and enjoy your Apple Cinnamon Oatmeal!

Scientific Note:

Rolled oats are a great source of complex carbohydrates and fiber, particularly beta-glucan, which can help lower cholesterol levels and stabilize blood sugar. Oats provide a slow release of energy, keeping you full longer and aiding in weight management.

Apples add natural sweetness and are rich in dietary fiber, which helps regulate digestion and maintain a feeling of fullness. They are also high in vitamins, especially vitamin C, which supports the immune system.

This recipe aligns with the Noom diet principles by offering a nutrient-dense, moderate-calorie meal that supports weight loss and overall well-being through the consumption of yellow-coded foods.

Nutritional Information (per serving):

- Calories: ~300
- Protein: 7g
- Total Fat: 10g
- Fiber: 6g
- Sodium: Low

Savory Sweet Potato Breakfast Bowl

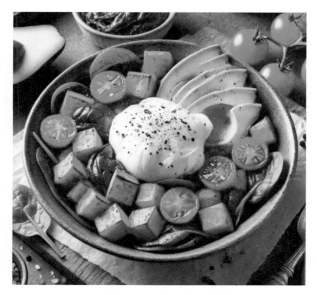

Serves: 1

Cooking Time: 20 minutes

Ingredients and Portions/Measurements:

- Sweet Potato (Noom diet yellow food friendly): 1 small, peeled and diced (Rich in vitamins A and C, provides fiber and complex carbohydrates)
- Olive Oil (Minimal amount for cooking): 1 teaspoon (Healthy fat, use sparingly)
- Egg (Noom diet yellow food friendly): 1 large, poached (High in protein, provides essential nutrients)
- Avocado (Noom diet yellow food friendly): 1/4 medium, sliced (Adds healthy fats and fiber)
- Cherry Tomatoes (Noom diet yellow food friendly): 1/4 cup, halved (Rich in vitamins A and C, low in calories)
- Spinach (Noom diet yellow food friendly): 1/2 cup, chopped (Rich in vitamins A, C, and K; low in calories)
- Salt and Black Pepper (Noom diet yellow food friendly): To taste (Adds flavor)

Instructions:

- Preheat the oven to 400°F (200°C).
- Toss the diced sweet potato with olive oil and spread evenly on a baking sheet. Roast in the oven for 15-20 minutes, or until tender and slightly crispy.

- While the sweet potato is roasting, poach the egg by bringing a small pot of water to a gentle simmer. Crack the egg into a small bowl and gently slide it into the simmering water. Cook for 3-4 minutes until the white is set but the yolk is still runny. Remove with a slotted spoon and set aside.
- In a small skillet, sauté the chopped spinach until wilted, about 2-3 minutes.
- Once the sweet potato is done, assemble the bowl by placing the roasted sweet potato at the bottom. Top with sautéed spinach, cherry tomatoes, and avocado slices.
- Place the poached egg on top and season with salt and black pepper to taste.
- Serve immediately and enjoy your Savory Sweet Potato Breakfast Bowl!

Scientific Note:

Sweet potatoes are an excellent source of complex carbohydrates, providing a slow release of energy that helps maintain blood sugar levels and keeps you feeling full longer. They are rich in vitamins A and C, which support immune function, skin health, and vision.

Eggs are a high-quality protein source and provide essential nutrients such as choline, which is important for brain health. Poaching eggs is a healthy cooking method that avoids adding extra fat.

Avocados add a creamy texture and are rich in monounsaturated fats, which are heart-healthy. They also provide fiber and essential nutrients like potassium and vitamins E and C.

This recipe aligns with the Noom diet principles by offering a nutrient-dense, moderate-calorie meal that supports weight loss and overall well-being through the consumption of yellow-coded foods.

Nutritional Information (per serving):

- Calories: ~320
- Protein: 10g
- Total Fat: 16g
- Fiber: 7g
- Sodium: Low

LUNCH RECIPES
YELLOW CODED FOODS

Mediterranean Quinoa Salad

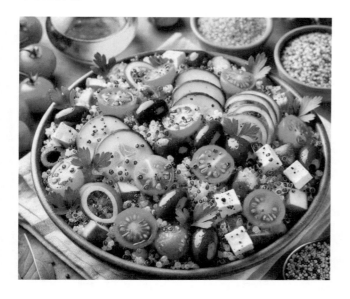

Serves: 1

Cooking Time: 20 minutes

Ingredients and Portions/Measurements:

- Quinoa (Noom diet yellow food friendly): 1/3 cup (Rich in protein, fiber, and essential amino acids; a healthy carb that's supportive of weight management)
- Water: 2/3 cup (For cooking quinoa)
- Cherry Tomatoes (Noom diet yellow food friendly): 1/2 cup, halved (Rich in vitamins A and C, low in calories)
- Cucumber (Noom diet yellow food friendly): 1/2 cup, diced (Hydrating and low in calories)
- Kalamata Olives (Noom diet yellow food friendly): 6 olives, sliced (Adds flavor and healthy fats)
- Feta Cheese (Substitute with vegan feta for dairy intolerance): 2 tablespoons, crumbled (Adds protein and calcium)
- Red Onion (Noom diet yellow food friendly): 2 tablespoons, finely chopped (Adds flavor and nutrients)
- Fresh Parsley (Noom diet yellow food friendly): 1 tablespoon, chopped (Adds flavor and nutrients)
- Olive Oil (Minimal amount for dressing): 1 teaspoon (Healthy fat, use sparingly)
- Lemon Juice (Noom diet yellow food friendly): 1 tablespoon (Adds flavor and vitamin C)
- Black Pepper (Noom diet yellow food friendly): To taste (Adds flavor without calories)

Instructions:

- Rinse the quinoa under cold water to remove its natural coating, saponin, which can make it taste bitter.
- In a small saucepan, bring water and quinoa to a boil. Reduce heat to low,

- cover, and simmer for 15 minutes or until the quinoa is tender and the water is absorbed.
- While the quinoa is cooking, prepare the vegetables: halve the cherry tomatoes, dice the cucumber, slice the olives, finely chop the red onion, and chop the fresh parsley.
- Once the quinoa is done, fluff it with a fork and let it cool for a few minutes.
- In a large bowl, combine the cooked quinoa, cherry tomatoes, cucumber, olives, feta cheese, red onion, and parsley.
- In a small bowl, whisk together the olive oil, lemon juice, and black pepper to make the dressing.
- Pour the dressing over the quinoa salad and toss gently to combine.
- Serve immediately and enjoy your Mediterranean Quinoa Salad!

Scientific Note:

Quinoa is a complete protein, providing all nine essential amino acids necessary for muscle repair and growth. It is also high in fiber, which aids in digestion and helps maintain a feeling of fullness, making it an excellent choice for weight management.

Feta cheese, though higher in calories, is used sparingly to add a creamy texture and a boost of protein and calcium. For those with dairy intolerance, vegan feta is a suitable alternative.

This recipe aligns with the Noom diet principles by offering a nutrient-dense, moderate-calorie meal that supports weight loss and overall well-being through the consumption of yellow-coded foods.

Nutritional Information (per serving):

- Calories: ~350
- Protein: 12g
- Total Fat: 15g
- Fiber: 5g
- Sodium: Moderate

Spicy Chickpea and Avocado Wrap

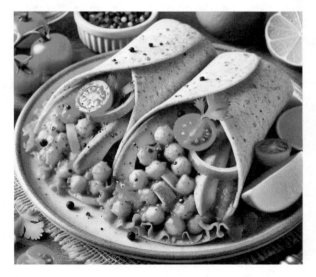

Serves: 1

Cooking Time: 10 minutes

Ingredients and Portions/Measurements:

- Whole Wheat Tortilla (Noom diet yellow food friendly): 1 medium (Rich in fiber, supports digestion)
- Chickpeas (Noom diet yellow food friendly): 1/4 cup, cooked and mashed (High in protein and fiber)
- Avocado (Noom diet yellow food friendly): 1/4 medium, sliced (Adds healthy fats and fiber)
- Cherry Tomatoes (Noom diet yellow food friendly): 1/4 cup, halved (Rich in vitamins A and C, low in calories)
- Red Onion (Noom diet yellow food friendly): 2 tablespoons, finely chopped (Adds flavor and nutrients)
- Fresh Cilantro (Noom diet yellow food friendly): 1 tablespoon, chopped (Adds flavor and nutrients)
- Lime Juice (Noom diet yellow food friendly): 1 tablespoon (Adds flavor and vitamin C)
- Hot Sauce (Noom diet yellow food friendly): 1 teaspoon (Optional, adds flavor and a spicy kick)
- Black Pepper (Noom diet yellow food friendly): To taste (Adds flavor without calories)

Instructions:

- In a bowl, mash the cooked chickpeas until mostly smooth, leaving some chunks for texture.
- Mix in the lime juice, chopped red onion, and black pepper. Add hot sauce if you prefer a spicy kick.
- Lay the whole wheat tortilla flat and spread the chickpea mixture evenly over the center.
- Layer the sliced avocado and halved cherry tomatoes on top of the chickpea mixture.
- Sprinkle with fresh cilantro.
- Roll up the tortilla tightly, folding in the sides as you go, to form a wrap.
- Serve immediately and enjoy your Spicy Chickpea and Avocado Wrap!

Scientific Note:

Whole wheat tortillas are a great source of dietary fiber, which aids in digestion and helps maintain a feeling of fullness. The fiber content also supports healthy blood sugar levels, making it a good choice for weight management.

Chickpeas are rich in protein and fiber, which help keep you full and satisfied. They also provide essential vitamins and minerals such as iron, magnesium, and folate, which support overall health and well-being.

Avocados add a creamy texture and are high in monounsaturated fats, which are heart-healthy. They also provide fiber, potassium, and vitamins E and C, which are beneficial for skin health and immune function.

Cherry tomatoes are packed with vitamins A and C, antioxidants that help protect the body from oxidative stress and support overall health. They are low in calories and high in fiber, adding bulk to meals without significantly increasing calorie intake.

This recipe aligns with the Noom diet principles by offering a nutrient-dense, moderate-calorie meal that supports weight loss and overall well-being through the consumption of yellow-coded foods.

Nutritional Information (per serving):

- Calories: ~320
- Protein: 10g
- Total Fat: 14g
- Fiber: 10g
- Sodium: Moderate

Lentil and Vegetable Stuffed Bell Pepper

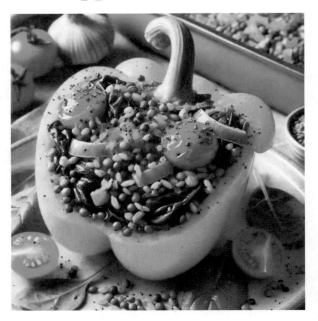

Serves: 1

Cooking Time: 25 minutes

Ingredients and Portions/Measurements:

- Bell Pepper (Noom diet yellow food friendly): 1 medium, halved and seeds removed (Rich in vitamins A and C, low in calories)
- Lentils (Noom diet yellow food friendly): 1/4 cup, cooked (High in protein and fiber)
- Brown Rice (Noom diet yellow food friendly): 1/4 cup, cooked (Provides fiber and complex carbohydrates)

- Cherry Tomatoes (Noom diet yellow food friendly): 1/4 cup, halved (Rich in vitamins A and C, low in calories)
- Spinach (Noom diet yellow food friendly): 1/2 cup, chopped (Rich in vitamins A, C, and K; low in calories)
- Olive Oil (Minimal amount for cooking): 1 teaspoon (Healthy fat, use sparingly)
- Red Onion (Noom diet yellow food friendly): 2 tablespoons, finely chopped (Adds flavor and nutrients)
- Garlic (Noom diet yellow food friendly): 1 clove, minced (Adds flavor and has health benefits)
- Black Pepper (Noom diet yellow food friendly): To taste (Adds flavor without calories)
- Fresh Parsley (Noom diet yellow food friendly): 1 tablespoon, chopped (Adds flavor and nutrients)
- Lemon Juice (Noom diet yellow food friendly): 1 teaspoon (Adds flavor and vitamin C)

Instructions:

- Preheat the oven to 375°F (190°C).
- Lightly spray a baking dish with olive oil.
- Place the halved bell pepper in the baking dish, cut side up.
- In a skillet, heat the olive oil over medium heat. Add the chopped red onion and minced garlic, sautéing until fragrant, about 2-3 minutes.
- Add the cooked lentils, brown rice, cherry tomatoes, and chopped spinach to the skillet. Cook for another 3-4 minutes until the spinach is wilted and the mixture is well combined.
- Season with black pepper and fresh parsley.
- Spoon the lentil and vegetable mixture into the bell pepper halves.
- Bake in the preheated oven for 15-20 minutes, or until the bell pepper is tender.
- Remove from the oven and drizzle with lemon juice before serving.
- Serve immediately and enjoy your Lentil and Vegetable Stuffed Bell Pepper!

Scientific Note:

Bell peppers are an excellent source of vitamins A and C, antioxidants that support immune function and skin health. They are low in calories and add bulk to meals without significantly increasing calorie intake.

Lentils are high in protein and fiber, which help keep you full and satisfied. They are also rich in essential nutrients such as iron, magnesium, and folate, which support overall health and well-being.

Brown rice provides complex carbohydrates and fiber, which aid in digestion and help maintain a feeling of fullness. The fiber content also supports healthy blood sugar levels, making it a good choice for weight management.

This recipe aligns with the Noom diet principles by offering a nutrient-dense, moderate-calorie meal that supports weight loss and overall well-being through the consumption of yellow-coded foods.

Nutritional Information (per serving):

- Calories: ~300
- Protein: 12g
- Total Fat: 5g
- Fiber: 10g
- Sodium: Low

Chicken and Avocado Salad Wrap

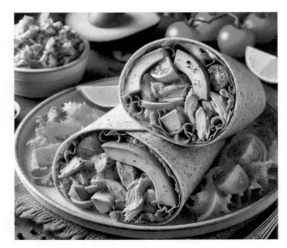

Serves: 1

Cooking Time: 15 minutes

Ingredients and Portions/Measurements:

- Whole Wheat Tortilla (Noom diet yellow food friendly): 1 medium (Rich in fiber, supports digestion)
- Cooked Chicken Breast (Noom diet yellow food friendly): 3 ounces, shredded (High in protein, low in fat)
- Avocado (Noom diet yellow food friendly): 1/4 medium, sliced (Adds healthy fats and fiber)
- Romaine Lettuce (Noom diet yellow food friendly): 1 cup, chopped (Low in calories, high in vitamins A and C)
- Cherry Tomatoes (Noom diet yellow food friendly): 1/4 cup, halved (Rich in vitamins A and C, low in calories)
- Red Onion (Noom diet yellow food friendly): 2 tablespoons, finely chopped (Adds flavor and nutrients)
- Fresh Cilantro (Noom diet yellow food friendly): 1 tablespoon, chopped (Adds flavor and nutrients)
- Lime Juice (Noom diet yellow food friendly): 1 tablespoon (Adds flavor and vitamin C)
- Olive Oil (Minimal amount for dressing): 1 teaspoon (Healthy fat, use sparingly)

- Black Pepper (Noom diet yellow food friendly): To taste (Adds flavor without calories)

Instructions:

- In a large bowl, combine the shredded chicken, sliced avocado, chopped romaine lettuce, halved cherry tomatoes, and finely chopped red onion.
- In a small bowl, whisk together the lime juice, olive oil, and black pepper to make the dressing.
- Pour the dressing over the chicken and vegetable mixture and toss gently to combine.
- Lay the whole wheat tortilla flat and spread the mixture evenly over the center.
- Sprinkle with fresh cilantro.
- Roll up the tortilla tightly, folding in the sides as you go, to form a wrap.
- Serve immediately and enjoy your Chicken and Avocado Salad Wrap!

Scientific Note:

Whole wheat tortillas are a great source of dietary fiber, which aids in digestion and helps maintain a feeling of fullness. The fiber content also supports healthy blood sugar levels, making it a good choice for weight management.

Chicken breast is high in protein and low in fat, making it an excellent choice for a lean protein source. Protein is essential for muscle repair and maintenance, and it helps keep you full longer.

Avocados add a creamy texture and are high in monounsaturated fats, which are heart-healthy. They also provide fiber, potassium, and vitamins E and C, which are beneficial for skin health and immune function.

Romaine lettuce is low in calories and high in vitamins A and C, supporting immune function and skin health. It also provides fiber, which aids in digestion.

This recipe aligns with the Noom diet principles by offering a nutrient-dense, moderate-calorie meal that supports weight loss and overall well-being through the consumption of yellow-coded foods.

Nutritional Information (per serving):

- Calories: ~320
- Protein: 22g
- Total Fat: 14g
- Fiber: 8g
- Sodium: Moderate

Tuna and Quinoa Salad

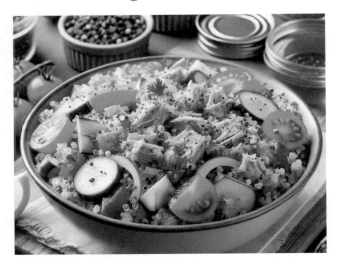

Serves: 1

Cooking Time: 20 minutes

Ingredients and Portions/Measurements:

- Quinoa (Noom diet yellow food friendly): 1/3 cup, cooked (Rich in protein, fiber, and essential amino acids)
- Canned Tuna in Water (Noom diet yellow food friendly): 1/2 can (about 2.5 ounces), drained (High in protein, low in fat)
- Cherry Tomatoes (Noom diet yellow food friendly): 1/4 cup, halved (Rich in vitamins A and C, low in calories)
- Cucumber (Noom diet yellow food friendly): 1/4 cup, diced (Hydrating and low in calories)

- Red Bell Pepper (Noom diet yellow food friendly): 1/4 cup, diced (Rich in vitamins A and C, low in calories)
- Red Onion (Noom diet yellow food friendly): 2 tablespoons, finely chopped (Adds flavor and nutrients)
- Fresh Parsley (Noom diet yellow food friendly): 1 tablespoon, chopped (Adds flavor and nutrients)
- Olive Oil (Minimal amount for dressing): 1 teaspoon (Healthy fat, use sparingly)
- Lemon Juice (Noom diet yellow food friendly): 1 tablespoon (Adds flavor and vitamin C)
- Black Pepper (Noom diet yellow food friendly): To taste (Adds flavor without calories)

Instructions:

- Cook the quinoa according to the package instructions and let it cool.
- In a large bowl, combine the cooked quinoa, drained tuna, halved cherry tomatoes, diced cucumber, diced red bell pepper, and finely chopped red onion.
- In a small bowl, whisk together the olive oil, lemon juice, and black pepper to make the dressing.
- Pour the dressing over the quinoa and tuna mixture and toss gently to combine.

- Sprinkle with fresh parsley.
- Serve immediately and enjoy your Tuna and Quinoa Salad!

Scientific Note:

Quinoa is a complete protein, providing all nine essential amino acids necessary for muscle repair and growth. It is also high in fiber, which aids in digestion and helps maintain a feeling of fullness, making it an excellent choice for weight management.

Tuna is an excellent source of lean protein, which is essential for muscle maintenance and repair. It is also rich in omega-3 fatty acids, which support heart health and reduce inflammation.

This recipe aligns with the Noom diet principles by offering a nutrient-dense, moderate-calorie meal that supports weight loss and overall well-being through the consumption of yellow-coded foods.

Nutritional Information (per serving):

- Calories: ~350
- Protein: 25g
- Total Fat: 10g
- Fiber: 6g
- Sodium: Moderate

DINNER RECIPES

(YELLOW CODED COLOR)

Lemon Herb Chicken with Quinoa

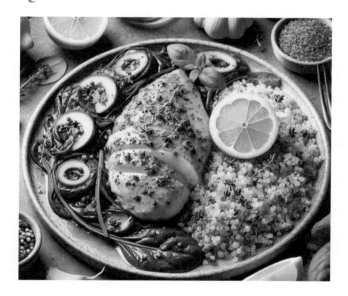

Serves: 1

Cooking Time: 30 minutes

Ingredients and Portions/Measurements:

- Chicken Breast (Yellow code color friendly): 1 medium (150g)
- Olive Oil (Yellow code color friendly): 1 tablespoon
- Lemon Juice (Yellow code color friendly): 1 tablespoon

- Garlic (Yellow code color friendly): 2 cloves, minced
- Fresh Rosemary (Yellow code color friendly): 1 teaspoon, chopped
- Fresh Thyme (Yellow code color friendly): 1 teaspoon, chopped
- Quinoa (Yellow code color friendly): 1/2 cup
- Water (For cooking quinoa): 1 cup
- Spinach (Yellow code color friendly): 1 cup
- Salt (Yellow code color friendly): to taste
- Black Pepper (Yellow code color friendly): to taste

Instructions:

- Preheat the oven to 375°F (190°C).
- In a small bowl, mix the olive oil, lemon juice, minced garlic, chopped rosemary, and chopped thyme.
- Season the chicken breast with salt and black pepper. Pour the lemon herb mixture over the chicken, ensuring it is well coated.
- Place the chicken in a baking dish and bake for 20-25 minutes or until the chicken is cooked through and the internal temperature reaches 165°F (74°C).
- While the chicken is baking, rinse the quinoa under cold water to remove its natural coating, saponin, which can make it taste bitter.
- In a medium saucepan, bring water to a boil. Add the quinoa, reduce the heat to low, cover, and simmer for 15 minutes or until the quinoa is tender and the water is absorbed. Fluff with a fork.
- In a large pan, wilt the spinach over medium heat for about 2-3 minutes until just cooked. Season with a pinch of salt and pepper.
- Serve the baked chicken breast over a bed of quinoa, with wilted spinach on the side. Garnish with a slice of lemon if desired.

Scientific Note:

Chicken breast is a lean source of protein that fits well within the yellow code color of the Noom diet. It's low in fat and calories while being rich in essential nutrients like B vitamins and selenium, which support overall metabolic health.

Quinoa, classified as a yellow food in the Noom diet, is a whole grain that provides a good balance of protein, fiber, and carbohydrates, making it a healthier carb choice that aids in sustained energy release and satiety.

Spinach, though green in color, is classified under yellow due to its nutrient density and low calorie content, offering vitamins A, C, and K, along with iron and calcium. Olive oil, used in moderation, is a healthy fat that supports heart health due to its monounsaturated fat content. This meal is balanced, nutrient-dense, and adheres to the yellow code color guidelines, promoting sustained energy and overall health.

Nutritional Information (per serving):

- Calories: ~420
- Protein: 35g
- Total Fat: 14g (mainly from olive oil)
- Fiber: 6g
- Sodium: moderate.

Spaghetti Squash with Tomato Basil Sauce

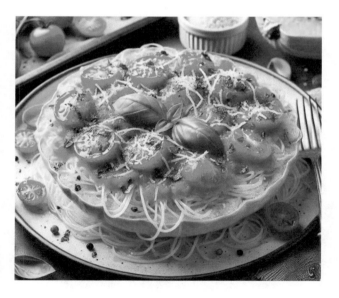

Serves: 1

Cooking Time: 40 minutes

Ingredients and Portions/Measurements:

- Spaghetti Squash (Yellow code color friendly): 1 small squash (about 2 cups cooked)
- Olive Oil (Yellow code color friendly): 1 tablespoon
- Cherry Tomatoes (Yellow code color friendly): 1 cup, halved
- Fresh Basil (Yellow code color friendly): 1/4 cup, chopped
- Garlic (Yellow code color friendly): 2 cloves, minced
- Onion (Yellow code color friendly): 1/4 cup, finely chopped
- Parmesan Cheese (Yellow code color friendly): 2 tablespoons, grated (optional)
- Salt (Yellow code color friendly): to taste
- Black Pepper (Yellow code color friendly): to taste

Instructions:

- Preheat the oven to 400°F (200°C). Cut the spaghetti squash in half lengthwise and scoop out the seeds. Drizzle with olive oil and season with salt and pepper. Place the squash halves cut-side down on a baking sheet and bake for 30-35 minutes, or until the squash is tender and easily shredded with a fork.

- While the squash is baking, heat 1 tablespoon of olive oil in a pan over medium heat. Add the chopped onion and minced garlic, cooking until the onion is translucent and the garlic is fragrant.
- Add the halved cherry tomatoes to the pan and cook until they start to break down and release their juices, about 5-7 minutes.
- Stir in the chopped basil, salt, and black pepper to taste. Let the sauce simmer for a few more minutes until it thickens slightly.
- Once the spaghetti squash is cooked, use a fork to scrape out the strands into a bowl.
- Pour the tomato basil sauce over the spaghetti squash and toss to combine.
- Top with grated Parmesan cheese if desired.
- Serve warm and enjoy your healthy, delicious dinner!

Scientific Note:

Spaghetti squash is a fantastic low-carb alternative to traditional pasta, making it a perfect yellow-coded food for the Noom diet. It is low in calories but high in fiber, which helps with digestion and keeping you full longer. Cherry tomatoes are rich in vitamins C and K, potassium, and folate, while also providing antioxidants like lycopene, which has been linked to many health benefits, including reduced risk of heart disease and cancer. Fresh basil adds flavor without added calories, and its essential oils have anti-inflammatory and antibacterial properties. Olive oil, used in moderation, provides healthy fats that support heart health. This recipe aligns with the Noom diet principles, offering a satisfying and nutritious meal that promotes overall well-being.

Nutritional Information (per serving):

- Calories: ~250
- Protein: 5g
- Total Fat: 12g (mainly from olive oil)
- Fiber: 7g
- Sodium: moderate

Chickpea and Vegetable Stir-Fry

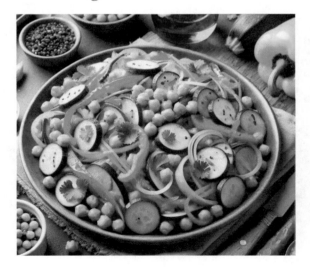

Serves: 1

Cooking Time: 25 minutes

Ingredients and Portions/Measurements:

- Chickpeas (Yellow code color friendly): 1 cup, cooked or canned (drained and rinsed)
- Olive Oil (Yellow code color friendly): 1 tablespoon
- Bell Pepper (Yellow code color friendly): 1/2 cup, sliced
- Zucchini (Yellow code color friendly): 1/2 cup, sliced
- Carrot (Yellow code color friendly): 1/2 cup, thinly sliced
- Onion (Yellow code color friendly): 1/4 cup, chopped
- Garlic (Yellow code color friendly): 2 cloves, minced
- Soy Sauce (Yellow code color friendly): 1 tablespoon (low sodium preferred)
- Fresh Ginger (Yellow code color friendly): 1 teaspoon, grated
- Fresh Cilantro (Yellow code color friendly): 2 tablespoons, chopped
- Lemon Juice (Yellow code color friendly): 1 tablespoon
- Salt (Yellow code color friendly): to taste
- Black Pepper (Yellow code color friendly): to taste

Instructions:

- Heat the olive oil in a large pan over medium heat. Add the chopped onion and minced garlic, cooking until the onion is translucent and the garlic is fragrant.
- Add the sliced bell pepper, zucchini, and carrot to the pan. Stir-fry for about 5-7 minutes until the vegetables are tender-crisp.
- Add the cooked chickpeas, soy sauce, and grated ginger to the pan. Stir well to combine all the ingredients.
- Cook for another 5 minutes, allowing the flavors to meld together. Stir occasionally.
- Add the lemon juice, chopped cilantro, salt, and black pepper. Stir to combine and cook for an additional minute.
- Serve hot and enjoy your nutritious and delicious chickpea and vegetable stir-fry!

Scientific Note:

Chickpeas are a great source of plant-based protein and fiber, making them a yellow-coded food in the Noom diet. They help in maintaining satiety and support digestive health. Bell peppers are rich in vitamins A and C, providing antioxidants that help protect cells from damage. Zucchini is low in calories but high in vitamins and minerals, including vitamin A, vitamin C, and potassium. Carrots are known for their high beta-carotene content, which the body converts to vitamin A, crucial for vision and immune function. Olive oil, used in moderation, provides healthy fats that support heart health. This meal is balanced, nutrient-dense, and adheres to the yellow code color guidelines, promoting sustained energy and overall health.

Nutritional Information (per serving):

- Calories: ~350
- Protein: 10g
- Total Fat: 12g (mainly from olive oil)
- Fiber: 12g
- Sodium: moderate

Baked Cod with Mango Salsa

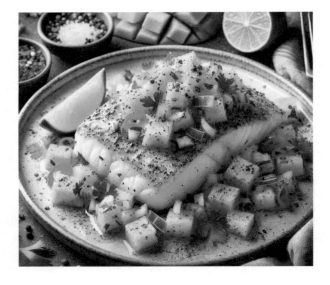

Serves: 1

Cooking Time: 30 minutes

Ingredients and Portions/Measurements:

- Cod Fillet (Yellow code color friendly): 1 fillet (about 150g)
- Olive Oil (Yellow code color friendly): 1 tablespoon
- Lime Juice (Yellow code color friendly): 1 tablespoon
- Garlic Powder (Yellow code color friendly): 1/2 teaspoon
- Paprika (Yellow code color friendly): 1/2 teaspoon
- Salt (Yellow code color friendly): to taste
- Black Pepper (Yellow code color friendly): to taste
- Mango Salsa:
- Mango (Yellow code color friendly): 1/2 cup, diced
- Red Onion (Yellow code color friendly): 1/4 cup, finely chopped
- Red Bell Pepper (Yellow code color friendly): 1/4 cup, diced
- Fresh Cilantro (Yellow code color friendly): 2 tablespoons, chopped
- Jalapeno (Yellow code color friendly): 1/2, finely chopped (optional)
- Lime Juice (Yellow code color friendly): 1 tablespoon
- Salt (Yellow code color friendly): to taste

Instructions:

- Preheat the oven to 400°F (200°C).

- In a small bowl, mix the olive oil, lime juice, garlic powder, paprika, salt, and black pepper.
- Place the cod fillet on a baking sheet lined with parchment paper. Brush the cod with the olive oil mixture.
- Bake the cod for 15-20 minutes or until the fish is opaque and flakes easily with a fork.
- While the cod is baking, prepare the mango salsa. In a medium bowl, combine the diced mango, red onion, red bell pepper, chopped cilantro, jalapeno (if using), lime juice, and salt. Mix well.
- Once the cod is done, remove it from the oven and let it rest for a couple of minutes.
- Serve the baked cod topped with the fresh mango salsa. Enjoy!

Scientific Note:

Cod is a lean protein source rich in vitamins B12 and B6, which are important for energy metabolism and maintaining healthy nerve function. It's a yellow-coded food in the Noom diet due to its low-calorie content and high protein density, aiding in muscle maintenance and repair.

Mango is high in vitamins A and C, supporting immune health and skin integrity. Red bell peppers are also rich in antioxidants like vitamin C, which helps reduce inflammation. The use of olive oil provides healthy monounsaturated fats, beneficial for heart health. This recipe offers a delightful balance of flavors and nutrients, adhering to the yellow code color guidelines of the Noom diet.

Nutritional Information (per serving):

- Calories: ~300
- Protein: 25g
- Total Fat: 10g (mainly from olive oil)
- Fiber: 4g
- Sodium: moderate

Moroccan-Spiced Lentil Stew

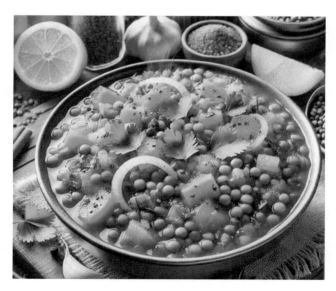

Serves: 1

Cooking Time: 35 minutes

Ingredients and Portions/Measurements:

- Lentils (Yellow code color friendly): 1/2 cup, dried
- Olive Oil (Yellow code color friendly): 1 tablespoon
- Onion (Yellow code color friendly): 1/4 cup, finely chopped
- Garlic (Yellow code color friendly): 2 cloves, minced
- Carrot (Yellow code color friendly): 1/2 cup, diced
- Celery (Yellow code color friendly): 1/2 cup, diced
- Canned Diced Tomatoes (Yellow code color friendly): 1/2 cup
- Vegetable Broth (Yellow code color friendly): 1 cup, low sodium
- Ground Cumin (Yellow code color friendly): 1/2 teaspoon
- Ground Coriander (Yellow code color friendly): 1/2 teaspoon
- Ground Cinnamon (Yellow code color friendly): 1/4 teaspoon
- Ground Ginger (Yellow code color friendly): 1/4 teaspoon
- Salt (Yellow code color friendly): to taste
- Black Pepper (Yellow code color friendly): to taste
- Fresh Cilantro (Yellow code color friendly): 2 tablespoons, chopped (for garnish)
- Lemon Wedges (Yellow code color friendly): for serving

Instructions:

- Rinse the lentils under cold water and set aside.
- In a large pot, heat the olive oil over medium heat. Add the chopped onion and minced garlic, cooking until the onion is translucent and the garlic is fragrant.
- Add the diced carrot and celery to the pot. Cook for about 5 minutes until the vegetables start to soften.
- Stir in the ground cumin, coriander, cinnamon, and ginger. Cook for 1 minute until the spices are fragrant.
- Add the rinsed lentils, canned diced tomatoes, and vegetable broth to the pot. Bring to a boil, then reduce the heat to low and simmer for about 25 minutes, or until the lentils are tender and the stew has thickened.
- Season with salt and black pepper to taste.
- Serve the stew hot, garnished with fresh cilantro and a squeeze of lemon juice from the lemon wedges.

Lentils are a fantastic source of plant-based protein and fiber, making them a yellow-coded food in the Noom diet. They support digestive health and help maintain satiety. The combination of spices, including cumin, coriander, cinnamon, and ginger, not only enhances the flavor but also provides anti-inflammatory and antioxidant benefits. Carrots and celery add vitamins A and K, as well as essential minerals like potassium. Olive oil, used in moderation, provides healthy monounsaturated fats that support heart health. This Moroccan-spiced lentil stew is a nutrient-dense, flavorful meal that aligns with the yellow code color guidelines of the Noom diet.

Nutritional Information (per serving):

- Calories: ˜350
- Protein: 15g
- Total Fat: 10g (mainly from olive oil)
- Fiber: 15g
- Sodium: 400mg

CHAPTER 4

BREAKFAST RECIPES

(RED CODED COLOUR)

Classic Pancake with Maple Syrup

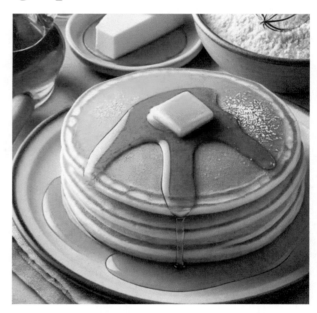

Serves: 1

Cooking Time: 15 minutes

Ingredients and Portions/Measurements:

- All-Purpose Flour (Noom diet red coded friendly): 1/3 cup (Provides carbohydrates and energy)

- Baking Powder (Noom diet red coded friendly): 1/2 teaspoon (Leavening agent)
- Sugar (Noom diet red coded friendly): 1 teaspoon (Adds sweetness)
- Salt (Noom diet red coded friendly): A pinch (Enhances flavor)
- Egg (Noom diet red coded friendly): 1 small (Provides protein and essential nutrients)
- Milk (Noom diet red coded friendly): 1/4 cup (Provides calcium and protein)
- Unsalted Butter (Noom diet red coded friendly): 1 tablespoon, melted (Adds richness and flavor)
- Pure Maple Syrup (Noom diet red coded friendly): 1 tablespoon (Natural sweetener)

Instructions:

- In a small bowl, whisk together the flour, baking powder, sugar, and salt.
- In another bowl, whisk the egg, milk, and melted butter until well combined.
- Add the wet ingredients to the dry ingredients and stir until just combined, being careful not to over mix.
- Heat a non-stick skillet or griddle over medium heat. Lightly grease with a small amount of butter or cooking spray.
- Pour the batter onto the skillet, using about 1/4 cup for each pancake.
- Cook until bubbles form on the surface of the pancake and the edges begin to look set, about 2-3 minutes. Flip and cook for an additional 1-2 minutes, or until golden brown.
- Serve the pancake immediately, drizzled with pure maple syrup.

Scientific Note:

All-purpose flour is a source of carbohydrates, which provide the body with energy. While it is considered a red-coded food in the Noom diet due to its refined nature, it can be enjoyed in moderation as part of a balanced diet.

Milk is a good source of calcium, vitamin D, and protein, all of which are important for bone health and overall body function. Using a small amount in this recipe adds nutritional value without significantly increasing calorie content.

Pure maple syrup, used sparingly, is a natural sweetener that contains antioxidants and minerals such as manganese and zinc. It adds sweetness and flavor to the pancakes without the need for refined sugars.

This recipe aligns with the Noom diet principles by providing a moderate-calorie breakfast that includes red-coded foods in a controlled portion. It emphasizes balance and moderation, allowing for the enjoyment of all foods within the context of a healthy diet.

Nutritional Information (per serving):

- Calories: ~250
- Protein: 6g
- Total Fat: 10g
- Fiber: 1g
- Sodium: Moderate

Sausage and Cheese Breakfast Muffin

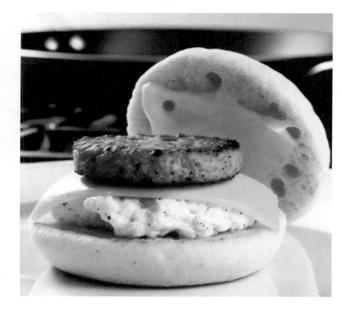

Serves: 1

Cooking Time: 25 minutes

Ingredients and Portions/Measurements:

- Breakfast Sausage (Noom diet red coded friendly): 1 small patty (High in protein, moderate in fat)
- Egg (Noom diet red coded friendly): 1 large (Provides protein and essential nutrients)
- Cheddar Cheese (Noom diet red coded friendly): 1/4 cup, shredded (Adds flavor and protein)
- English Muffin (Noom diet red coded friendly): 1 whole (Provides carbohydrates and energy)
- Butter (Noom diet red coded friendly): 1 teaspoon (Adds richness and flavor)
- Salt (Noom diet red coded friendly): A pinch (Enhances flavor)
- Black Pepper (Noom diet red coded friendly): To taste (Adds flavor without calories)

Instructions:

- Preheat the oven to 375°F (190°C).
- Cook the sausage patty in a non-stick skillet over medium heat until fully cooked, about 5-7 minutes per side. Remove from heat and set aside.
- In the same skillet, lightly scramble the egg, seasoning with a pinch of salt and black pepper. Cook until set, about 2-3 minutes.

- Split the English muffin in half and toast until golden brown.
- Spread the butter evenly on both halves of the toasted English muffin.
- Assemble the muffin by placing the sausage patty on the bottom half, followed by the scrambled egg, and then sprinkle the shredded cheddar cheese on top.
- Place the muffin halves on a baking sheet and bake in the preheated oven for about 5 minutes, or until the cheese is melted.
- Remove from the oven, assemble the sandwich, and serve immediately.

Scientific Note:

Breakfast sausage is a high-protein food that provides essential amino acids necessary for muscle repair and growth. However, it is also higher in fat and sodium, which is why it is classified as a red-coded food in the Noom diet. Consuming it in moderation as part of a balanced diet can help maintain energy levels and support muscle health.

Eggs are an excellent source of high-quality protein and provide important nutrients such as choline, which is crucial for brain health. The protein content helps keep you full and supports muscle maintenance and repair.

Cheddar cheese adds flavor and protein to the meal. It is also a good source of calcium and vitamin D, which are important for bone health. However, due to its higher fat content, it is classified as a red-coded food and should be consumed in moderation.

An English muffin provides carbohydrates, which are the body's primary source of energy. While it is considered a red-coded food due to its refined nature, it can be enjoyed in controlled portions as part of a balanced diet.

This recipe aligns with the Noom diet principles by providing a nutrient-dense, moderate-calorie breakfast that includes red-coded foods in a controlled portion. It emphasizes balance and moderation, allowing for the enjoyment of all foods within the context of a healthy diet.

Nutritional Information (per serving):

- Calories: ~400
- Protein: 20g
- Total Fat: 25g
- Fiber: 2g
- Sodium: Moderate

Bacon and Egg Breakfast Wrap

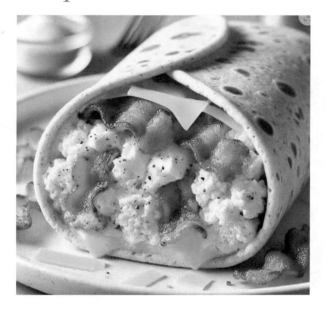

Serves: 1

Cooking Time: 15 minutes

Ingredients and Portions/Measurements:

- Bacon (Noom diet red coded friendly): 2 slices, cooked and crumbled (High in protein and fat)
- Egg (Noom diet red coded friendly): 1 large, scrambled (Provides protein and essential nutrients)
- Cheddar Cheese (Noom diet red coded friendly): 1/4 cup, shredded (Adds flavor and protein)
- Whole Wheat Tortilla (Noom diet red coded friendly): 1 medium (Provides carbohydrates and fiber)
- Butter (Noom diet red coded friendly): 1 teaspoon (Adds richness and flavor)
- Salt (Noom diet red coded friendly): A pinch (Enhances flavor)
- Black Pepper (Noom diet red coded friendly): To taste (Adds flavor without calories)

Instructions:

- Cook the bacon in a non-stick skillet over medium heat until crispy. Remove and place on a paper towel to drain excess fat. Once cooled, crumble the bacon.
- In the same skillet, scramble the egg with a pinch of salt and black pepper until fully cooked, about 2-3 minutes.
- Warm the whole wheat tortilla in the microwave or on a skillet for about 10-15 seconds until pliable.
- Spread the butter evenly on one side of the tortilla.
- Place the scrambled egg in the center of the tortilla. Sprinkle the shredded cheddar cheese over the egg and add the crumbled bacon.
- Roll up the tortilla, folding in the sides as you go to form a wrap.
- Serve immediately and enjoy your Bacon and Egg Breakfast Wrap!

Scientific Note:

Bacon is a high-protein food that provides essential amino acids necessary for muscle repair and growth. However, it is also high in fat and sodium, which is why it is classified as a red-coded food in the Noom diet. Consuming it in moderation as part of a balanced diet can help maintain energy levels and support muscle health.

A whole wheat tortilla provides carbohydrates and fiber, which aid in digestion and help maintain a feeling of fullness. While it is considered a red-coded food due to its refined nature, it can be enjoyed in controlled portions as part of a balanced diet.

This recipe aligns with the Noom diet principles by providing a nutrient-dense, moderate-calorie breakfast that includes red-coded foods in a controlled portion. It emphasizes balance and moderation, allowing for the enjoyment of all foods within the context of a healthy diet.

Nutritional Information (per serving):

- Calories: ~350
- Protein: 20g
- Total Fat: 22g
- Fiber: 4g
- Sodium: Moderate

Sausage and Cheese Breakfast Burrito

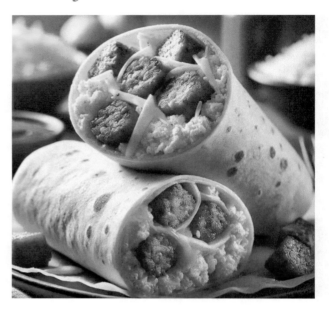

Serves: 1

Cooking Time: 20 minutes

Ingredients and Portions/Measurements:

- Pork Sausage (Noom diet red coded friendly): 2 ounces, cooked and crumbled (High in protein and fat)
- Egg (Noom diet red coded friendly): 1 large, scrambled (Provides protein and essential nutrients)
- Cheddar Cheese (Noom diet red coded friendly): 1/4 cup, shredded (Adds flavor and protein)
- White Flour Tortilla (Noom diet red coded friendly): 1 medium (Provides carbohydrates and energy)

- Butter (Noom diet red coded friendly): 1 teaspoon (Adds richness and flavor)
- Salt (Noom diet red coded friendly): A pinch (Enhances flavor)
- Black Pepper (Noom diet red coded friendly): To taste (Adds flavor without calories)
- Hot Sauce (Optional, for flavor): 1 teaspoon (Adds flavor and spice)

Instructions:

- Cook the pork sausage in a non-stick skillet over medium heat until fully cooked and browned, about 5-7 minutes. Remove and set aside.
- In the same skillet, scramble the egg with a pinch of salt and black pepper until fully cooked, about 2-3 minutes.
- Warm the white flour tortilla in the microwave or on a skillet for about 10-15 seconds until pliable.
- Spread the butter evenly on one side of the tortilla.
- Place the scrambled egg in the center of the tortilla. Sprinkle the shredded cheddar cheese over the egg and add the cooked sausage.
- Add hot sauce if desired for extra flavor.
- Roll up the tortilla, folding in the sides as you go to form a burrito.

- Serve immediately and enjoy your Sausage and Cheese Breakfast Burrito!

Scientific Note:

Pork sausage is a high-protein food that provides essential amino acids necessary for muscle repair and growth. However, it is also high in fat and sodium, which is why it is classified as a red-coded food in the Noom diet. Consuming it in moderation as part of a balanced diet can help maintain energy levels and support muscle health.

A white flour tortilla provides carbohydrates, which are the body's primary source of energy. While it is considered a red-coded food due to its refined nature, it can be enjoyed in controlled portions as part of a balanced diet.

This recipe aligns with the Noom diet principles by providing a nutrient-dense, moderate-calorie breakfast that includes red-coded foods in a controlled portion. It emphasizes balance and moderation, allowing for the enjoyment of all foods within the context of a healthy diet.

Nutritional Information (per serving):

- Calories: ~400
- Protein: 22g
- Total Fat: 26g
- Fiber: 2g
- Sodium: Moderate

Ham and Cheese Omelette

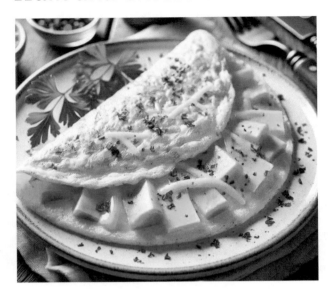

Serves: 1

Cooking Time: 15 minutes

Ingredients and Portions/Measurements:

- Ham (Noom diet red coded friendly): 2 ounces, diced (High in protein, moderate in fat)
- Egg (Noom diet red coded friendly): 2 large (Provides protein and essential nutrients)
- Cheddar Cheese (Noom diet red coded friendly): 1/4 cup, shredded (Adds flavor and protein)
- Butter (Noom diet red coded friendly): 1 teaspoon (Adds richness and flavor)
- Salt (Noom diet red coded friendly): A pinch (Enhances flavor)
- Black Pepper (Noom diet red coded friendly): To taste (Adds flavor without calories)
- Fresh Parsley (Optional, for garnish): 1 tablespoon, chopped (Adds flavor and nutrients)

Instructions:

- In a small bowl, whisk the eggs with a pinch of salt and black pepper until well combined.
- Heat the butter in a non-stick skillet over medium heat until melted.
- Pour the egg mixture into the skillet, tilting the pan to spread it evenly.
- As the eggs begin to set, sprinkle the diced ham and shredded cheddar cheese over one half of the omelette.
- Cook for another 1-2 minutes until the cheese begins to melt.
- Fold the other half of the omelette over the filling.
- Slide the omelette onto a plate and garnish with fresh parsley if desired.
- Serve immediately and enjoy your Ham and Cheese Omelette!

Scientific Note:

Ham is a high-protein food that provides essential amino acids necessary for muscle repair and growth. However, it is also high in sodium, which is why it is classified as a red-coded food in the Noom diet. Consuming it in moderation as part of a balanced diet can help maintain energy levels and support muscle health.

Butter, while adding richness and flavor, is also high in saturated fat and should be used sparingly. It is included in this recipe in a minimal amount to enhance the taste without significantly increasing the calorie content.

This recipe aligns with the Noom diet principles by providing a nutrient-dense, moderate-calorie breakfast that includes red-coded foods in a controlled portion. It emphasizes balance and moderation, allowing for the enjoyment of all foods within the context of a healthy diet.

Nutritional Information (per serving):

- Calories: ~350
- Protein: 24g
- Total Fat: 26g
- Fiber: 1g

LUNCH RECIPES

RED CODED COLOR

BBQ Chicken Wrap

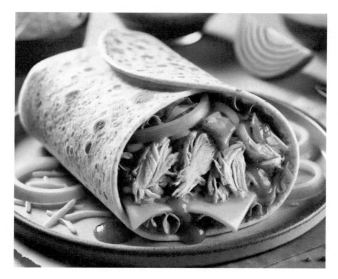

Serves: 1

Cooking Time: 20 minutes

Ingredients and Portions/Measurements:

- BBQ Chicken Breast (Noom diet red coded friendly): 3 ounces, shredded (High in protein, moderate in fat)
- Whole Wheat Tortilla (Noom diet red coded friendly): 1 medium (Provides carbohydrates and fiber)
- Cheddar Cheese (Noom diet red coded friendly): 1/4 cup, shredded (Adds flavor and protein)

- BBQ Sauce (Noom diet red coded friendly): 1 tablespoon (Adds flavor)
- Red Onion (Optional): 2 tablespoons, thinly sliced (Adds flavor and nutrients)
- Romaine Lettuce (Optional): 1/2 cup, shredded (Adds crunch and nutrients)
- Olive Oil (Minimal amount for cooking): 1 teaspoon (Healthy fat, use sparingly)
- Salt (Noom diet red coded friendly): A pinch (Enhances flavor)
- Black Pepper (Noom diet red coded friendly): To taste (Adds flavor without calories)

Instructions:

- Heat the olive oil in a non-stick skillet over medium heat.
- Add the shredded BBQ chicken breast to the skillet. Cook for about 3-4 minutes until heated through.
- Warm the whole wheat tortilla in the microwave or on a skillet for about 10-15 seconds until pliable.
- Place the warmed tortilla on a flat surface. Spread the BBQ sauce evenly over the tortilla.
- Layer the shredded BBQ chicken in the center of the tortilla.
- Sprinkle the shredded cheddar cheese over the chicken.
- Add thinly sliced red onion and shredded romaine lettuce if desired.
- Season with a pinch of salt and black pepper to taste.
- Roll up the tortilla, folding in the sides as you go to form a wrap.
- Serve immediately and enjoy your BBQ Chicken Wrap!

Scientific Note:

BBQ chicken breast is a high-protein food that provides essential amino acids necessary for muscle repair and growth. However, it is also moderate in sodium due to the BBQ sauce, which is why it is classified as a red-coded food in the Noom diet. Consuming it in moderation as part of a balanced diet can help maintain energy levels and support muscle health.

A whole wheat tortilla provides carbohydrates and fiber, which aid in digestion and help maintain a feeling of fullness. While it is considered a red-coded food due to its refined nature, it can be enjoyed in controlled portions as part of a balanced diet.

This recipe aligns with the Noom diet principles by providing a nutrient-dense, moderate-calorie lunch that includes red-coded foods in a controlled portion. It emphasizes balance and moderation, allowing for the enjoyment of all foods within the context of a healthy diet.

Nutritional Information (per serving):

- Calories: ~400
- Protein: 28g
- Total Fat: 18g
- Fiber: 4g
- Sodium: Moderate

Beef and Cheese Quesadilla

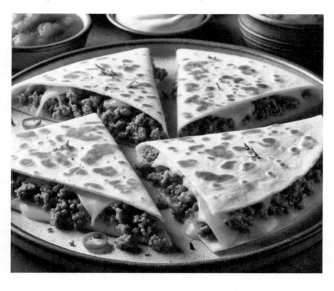

Serves: 1

Cooking Time: 20 minutes

Ingredients and Portions/Measurements:

- Ground Beef (Noom diet red coded friendly): 3 ounces, cooked and crumbled (High in protein, moderate in fat)
- Cheddar Cheese (Noom diet red coded friendly): 1/4 cup, shredded (Adds flavor and protein)
- Flour Tortilla (Noom diet red coded friendly): 1 medium (Provides carbohydrates and fiber)
- Olive Oil (Minimal amount for cooking): 1 teaspoon (Healthy fat, use sparingly)
- Salt (Noom diet red coded friendly): A pinch (Enhances flavor)
- Black Pepper (Noom diet red coded friendly): To taste (Adds flavor without calories)
- Salsa (Optional, for serving): 2 tablespoons (Adds flavor and moisture)
- Sour Cream (Optional, for serving): 1 tablespoon (Adds richness and flavor)

Instructions:

- Heat a non-stick skillet over medium heat and add the olive oil.
- Add the cooked and crumbled ground beef to the skillet. Season with a pinch of salt and black pepper. Cook for about 3-4 minutes until heated through.
- Remove the beef from the skillet and set aside.
- Wipe the skillet clean and place the flour tortilla in the skillet over medium heat.
- Sprinkle half of the shredded cheddar cheese evenly over one half of the tortilla.
- Spread the cooked ground beef over the cheese layer.

- Sprinkle the remaining cheddar cheese over the beef.
- Fold the tortilla in half to cover the filling.
- Cook for about 2-3 minutes on each side, or until the tortilla is golden brown and the cheese is melted.
- Remove from the skillet and cut into wedges.
- Serve immediately with salsa and sour cream on the side if desired.

Scientific Note:

Ground beef is a high-protein food that provides essential amino acids necessary for muscle repair and growth. However, it is also moderate in fat and should be consumed in moderation as part of a balanced diet.

Cheddar cheese adds flavor and protein to the meal. It is also a good source of calcium and vitamin D, which are important for bone health. However, due to its higher fat content, it is classified as a red-coded food and should be consumed in moderation.

A flour tortilla provides carbohydrates, which are the body's primary source of energy. While it is considered a red-coded food due to its refined nature, it can be enjoyed in controlled portions as part of a balanced diet.

This recipe aligns with the Noom diet principles by providing a nutrient-dense, moderate-calorie lunch that includes red-coded foods in a controlled portion. It emphasizes balance and moderation, allowing for the enjoyment of all foods within the context of a healthy diet.

Nutritional Information (per serving):

- Calories: ~450
- Protein: 26g
- Total Fat: 25g
- Fiber: 2g
- Sodium: Moderate

Ham and Swiss Cheese Panini

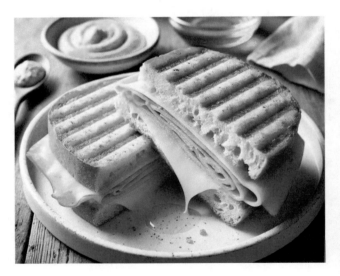

Serves: 1

Cooking Time: 15 minutes

Ingredients and Portions/Measurements:

- Sliced Ham (Noom diet red coded friendly): 3 ounces (High in protein, moderate in fat)
- Swiss Cheese (Noom diet red coded friendly): 2 slices (Adds flavor and protein)
- Sourdough Bread (Noom diet red coded friendly): 2 slices (Provides carbohydrates and fiber)
- Butter (Noom diet red coded friendly): 1 teaspoon (Adds richness and flavor)
- Dijon Mustard (Optional): 1 teaspoon (Adds flavor)
- Olive Oil (Minimal amount for cooking): 1 teaspoon (Healthy fat, use sparingly)

Instructions:

- Heat a panini press or non-stick skillet over medium heat.
- Spread the Dijon mustard on one side of each slice of sourdough bread (optional).
- Layer the sliced ham and Swiss cheese between the slices of bread to make a sandwich.
- Lightly spread butter on the outer sides of the sandwich.
- Place the sandwich on the panini press or skillet. If using a skillet, press down with a spatula.
- Cook for about 3-4 minutes on each side, or until the bread is golden brown and the cheese is melted.
- Remove from heat, cut in half, and serve immediately.

Scientific Note:

Ham is a high-protein food that provides essential *amino acids necessary for muscle repair and growth. However, it is also high in sodium, which is why it is classified as a red-coded food in the Noom diet. Consuming it in moderation as part of a balanced diet can help maintain energy levels and support muscle health.*

Swiss cheese adds flavor and protein to the meal. It is also a good source of calcium and vitamin D, which are important for bone health. However, due to its higher fat content, it is classified as a red-coded food and should be consumed in moderation.

Sourdough bread provides carbohydrates, which are the body's primary source of energy. While it is considered a red-coded food due to its refined nature, it can be enjoyed in controlled portions as part of a balanced diet.

This recipe aligns with the Noom diet principles by providing a nutrient-dense, moderate-calorie lunch that includes red-coded foods in a controlled portion. It emphasizes balance and moderation, allowing for the enjoyment of all foods within the context of a healthy diet.

Nutritional Information (per serving):

- Calories: ~450
- Protein: 28g
- Total Fat: 22g
- Fiber: 3g
- Sodium: Moderate

Spicy Beef and Cheese Wrap

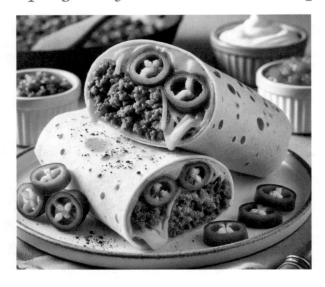

Serves: 1

Cooking Time: 20 minutes

Ingredients and Portions/Measurements:

- Ground Beef (Noom diet red coded friendly): 3 ounces (High in protein, moderate in fat)

- Cheddar Cheese (Noom diet red coded friendly): 1/4 cup, shredded (Adds flavor and protein)

- White Flour Tortilla (Noom diet red coded friendly): 1 medium (Provides carbohydrates and energy)

- Olive Oil (Minimal amount for cooking): 1 teaspoon (Healthy fat, use sparingly)

- Jalapeño (Optional, for spice): 1 small, sliced (Adds flavor and spice)

- Salsa (Optional, for serving): 2 tablespoons (Adds flavor and moisture)

- Sour Cream (Optional, for serving): 1 tablespoon (Adds richness and flavor)

- Salt (Noom diet red coded friendly): A pinch (Enhances flavor)

- Black Pepper (Noom diet red coded friendly): To taste (Adds flavor without calories)

Instructions:

- Heat the olive oil in a non-stick skillet over medium heat.

- Add the ground beef to the skillet. Season with a pinch of salt and black pepper. Cook for about 5-7 minutes until browned and fully cooked.

- Remove the beef from the skillet and set aside.

- In the same skillet, lightly warm the flour tortilla for about 10-15 seconds on each side until pliable.
- Place the tortilla on a flat surface. Spread the cooked ground beef evenly over the center of the tortilla.
- Sprinkle the shredded cheddar cheese over the beef.
- Add sliced jalapeño if desired for extra spice.
- Roll up the tortilla, folding in the sides as you go to form a wrap.
- Return the wrap to the skillet and cook for about 2-3 minutes on each side until the tortilla is golden brown and the cheese is melted.
- Serve immediately with salsa and sour cream on the side if desired.

Scientific Note:

Ground beef is a high-protein food that provides essential amino acids necessary for muscle repair and growth. However, it is also moderate in fat and should be consumed in moderation as part of a balanced diet.

A white flour tortilla provides carbohydrates, which are the body's primary source of energy. While it is considered a red-coded food due to its refined nature, it can be enjoyed in controlled portions as part of a balanced diet.

This recipe aligns with the Noom diet principles by providing a nutrient-dense, moderate-calorie lunch that includes red-coded foods in a controlled portion. It emphasizes balance and moderation, allowing for the enjoyment of all foods within the context of a healthy diet.

Nutritional Information (per serving):

- Calories: ~450
- Protein: 26g
- Total Fat: 25g
- Fiber: 2g
- Sodium: Moderate

Classic Bacon and Avocado Sandwich

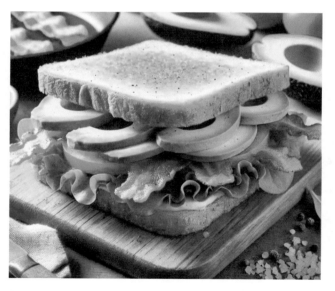

Serves: 1

Cooking Time: 15 minutes

Ingredients and Portions/Measurements:

- Bacon (Noom diet red coded friendly): 2 slices, cooked (High in protein and fat)
- Avocado (Noom diet red coded friendly): 1/2 medium, sliced (Adds healthy fats and fiber)
- Whole Wheat Bread (Noom diet red coded friendly): 2 slices (Provides carbohydrates and fiber)
- Mayonnaise (Noom diet red coded friendly): 1 teaspoon (Adds richness and flavor)
- Tomato (Noom diet red coded friendly): 2 slices (Adds vitamins and flavor)
- Lettuce (Noom diet red coded friendly): 2 leaves (Adds crunch and nutrients)
- Salt (Noom diet red coded friendly): A pinch (Enhances flavor)
- Black Pepper (Noom diet red coded friendly): To taste (Adds flavor without calories)

Instructions:

- Cook the bacon in a non-stick skillet over medium heat until crispy. Remove and place on a paper towel to drain excess fat.
- While the bacon is cooking, toast the whole wheat bread slices until golden brown.
- Spread the mayonnaise evenly on one side of each toast slice.
- Layer the lettuce leaves on one slice of the toasted bread.
- Add the tomato slices and then the avocado slices on top of the lettuce.
- Place the crispy bacon slices on top of the avocado.
- Season with a pinch of salt and black pepper to taste.
- Top with the second slice of toast, mayonnaise side down.
- Cut the sandwich in half and serve immediately.

Scientific Note:

Bacon is a high-protein food that provides essential amino acids necessary for muscle repair and growth. However, it is also high in fat and sodium, which is why it is classified as a red-coded food in the Noom diet. Consuming it in moderation as part of a balanced diet can help maintain energy levels and support muscle health.

Whole wheat bread provides carbohydrates and fiber, which aid in digestion and help maintain a feeling of fullness. While it is considered a red-coded food due to its refined nature, it can be enjoyed in controlled portions as part of a balanced diet.

This recipe aligns with the Noom diet principles by providing a nutrient-dense, moderate-calorie lunch that includes red-coded foods in a controlled portion. It emphasizes balance and moderation, allowing for the enjoyment of all foods within the context of a healthy diet.

Nutritional Information (per serving):

- Calories: ~450
- Protein: 15g
- Total Fat: 30g
- Fiber: 8g
- Sodium: Moderate

DINNER RECIPES

RED CODED COLOR

Grilled Steak with Garlic Butter

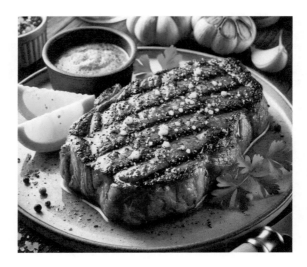

Serves: 1

Cooking Time: 25 minutes

Ingredients and Portions/Measurements:

- Sirloin Steak (Noom diet red coded friendly): 6 ounces (High in protein, moderate in fat)
- Butter (Noom diet red coded friendly): 1 tablespoon (Adds richness and flavor)
- Garlic (Noom diet red coded friendly): 2 cloves, minced (Adds flavor and has health benefits)

- Olive Oil (Minimal amount for cooking): 1 teaspoon (Healthy fat, use sparingly)
- Salt (Noom diet red coded friendly): A pinch (Enhances flavor)
- Black Pepper (Noom diet red coded friendly): To taste (Adds flavor without calories)
- Fresh Parsley (Optional, for garnish): 1 tablespoon, chopped (Adds flavor and nutrients)
- Lemon Wedges (Optional, for serving): 2 wedges (Adds flavor and vitamin C)

Instructions:

- Preheat the grill to medium-high heat.
- Season the sirloin steak with salt and black pepper on both sides.
- In a small saucepan, melt the butter over medium heat. Add the minced garlic and cook for about 2 minutes until fragrant. Remove from heat and set aside.
- Brush the steak with olive oil to prevent sticking.
- Place the steak on the grill and cook for about 4-5 minutes per side, or until it reaches your desired level of doneness.
- Remove the steak from the grill and let it rest for a few minutes.
- Drizzle the garlic butter over the steak.
- Garnish with fresh parsley and serve with lemon wedges if desired.
- Enjoy your Grilled Steak with Garlic Butter immediately!

Scientific Note:

Sirloin steak is a high-protein food that provides essential amino acids necessary for muscle repair and growth. However, it is also moderate in fat and should be consumed in moderation as part of a balanced diet. Protein helps maintain muscle mass and supports overall body functions.

Butter adds richness and flavor to the dish. While it is high in saturated fat, using it sparingly can enhance the taste without significantly increasing calorie content. It should be consumed in moderation as part of a balanced diet.

Garlic not only enhances the flavor of the dish but also provides numerous health benefits. It has anti-inflammatory and antioxidant properties and supports heart health.

This recipe aligns with the Noom diet principles by providing a nutrient-dense, moderate-calorie dinner that includes red-coded foods in a controlled portion. It emphasizes balance and moderation, allowing for the enjoyment of all foods within the context of a healthy diet.

Nutritional Information (per serving):

- Calories: ~450
- Protein: 38g
- Total Fat: 30g
- Fiber: 0g
- Sodium: Moderate

Pork Chop with Apple Glaze

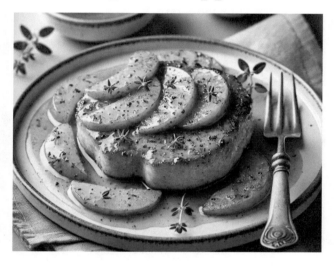

Serves: 1

Cooking Time: 30 minutes

Ingredients and Portions/Measurements:

- Pork Chop (Noom diet red coded friendly): 6 ounces (High in protein, moderate in fat)
- Olive Oil (Minimal amount for cooking): 1 teaspoon (Healthy fat, use sparingly)
- Apple Cider Vinegar (Noom diet red coded friendly): 1 tablespoon (Adds tangy flavor)
- Apple (Noom diet red coded friendly): 1 small, thinly sliced (Adds natural sweetness)
- Brown Sugar (Noom diet red coded friendly): 1 teaspoon (Adds sweetness)
- Salt (Noom diet red coded friendly): A pinch (Enhances flavor)
- Black Pepper (Noom diet red coded friendly): To taste (Adds flavor without calories)
- Fresh Thyme (Optional, for garnish): 1 teaspoon (Adds flavor and nutrients)

Instructions:

- Preheat the oven to 375°F (190°C).
- Season the pork chop with salt and black pepper on both sides.
- Heat the olive oil in a skillet over medium-high heat.
- Add the pork chop to the skillet and sear for about 3-4 minutes on each side until browned.
- Remove the pork chop from the skillet and place it on a baking sheet. Bake in the preheated oven for about 20 minutes, or until the internal temperature reaches 145°F (63°C).

- In the same skillet, add the apple cider vinegar, apple slices, and brown sugar. Cook over medium heat, stirring occasionally, until the apples are soft and the sauce is slightly thickened, about 5-7 minutes.
- Remove the pork chop from the oven and let it rest for a few minutes.
- Spoon the apple glaze over the pork chop.
- Garnish with fresh thyme if desired.
- Serve immediately and enjoy your Pork Chop with Apple Glaze!

Scientific Note:

Pork chops are a high-protein food that provides essential amino acids necessary for muscle repair and growth. However, they are also moderate in fat and should be consumed in moderation as part of a balanced diet. Protein helps maintain muscle mass and supports overall body functions.

Apples add natural sweetness and fiber to the dish. They are rich in vitamins and antioxidants, which support immune function and overall health. The fiber content helps with digestion and promotes satiety.

This recipe aligns with the Noom diet principles by providing a nutrient-dense, moderate-calorie dinner that includes red-coded foods in a controlled portion. It emphasizes balance and moderation, allowing for the enjoyment of all foods within the context of a healthy diet.

Nutritional Information (per serving):

- Calories: ~450
- Protein: 32g
- Total Fat: 22g
- Fiber: 3g
- Sodium: Moderate

Classic Turkey Club Sandwich

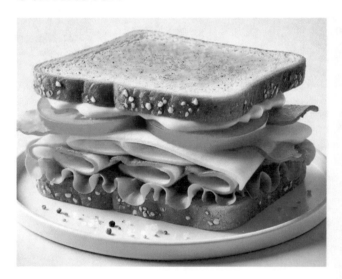

Serves: 1

Cooking Time: 15 minutes

Ingredients and Portions/Measurements:

- Sliced Turkey Breast (Noom diet red coded friendly): 3 ounces (High in protein, low in fat)

- Bacon (Noom diet red coded friendly): 2 slices, cooked (High in protein, moderate in fat)
- Whole Wheat Bread (Noom diet red coded friendly): 2 slices (Provides carbohydrates and fiber)
- Mayonnaise (Noom diet red coded friendly): 1 tablespoon (Adds richness and flavor)
- Tomato (Noom diet red coded friendly): 2 slices (Adds vitamins and flavor)
- Romaine Lettuce (Noom diet red coded friendly): 2 leaves (Adds crunch and nutrients)
- Salt (Noom diet red coded friendly): A pinch (Enhances flavor)
- Black Pepper (Noom diet red coded friendly): To taste (Adds flavor without calories)

Instructions:

- Toast the whole wheat bread slices until golden brown.
- Spread the mayonnaise evenly on one side of each slice of toasted bread.
- Layer the romaine lettuce leaves on one slice of the toasted bread.
- Add the sliced turkey breast on top of the lettuce.
- Place the cooked bacon slices on top of the turkey.
- Add the tomato slices on top of the bacon.
- Season with a pinch of salt and black pepper to taste.
- Top with the second slice of toasted bread, mayonnaise side down.
- Cut the sandwich in half and serve immediately.

Scientific Note:

Turkey breast is a high-protein, low-fat food that provides essential amino acids necessary for muscle repair and growth. Protein helps maintain muscle mass and supports overall body functions.

Bacon, while high in protein, is also moderate in fat and should be consumed in moderation as part of a balanced diet. It adds flavor and texture to the sandwich.

This recipe aligns with the Noom diet principles by providing a nutrient-dense, moderate-calorie lunch that includes red-coded foods in a controlled portion. It emphasizes balance and moderation, allowing for the enjoyment of all foods within the context of a healthy diet.

Nutritional Information (per serving):

- Calories: ~400
- Protein: 28g
- Total Fat: 20g

- Fiber: 5g
- Sodium: Moderate

Beef Stroganoff with Mushrooms

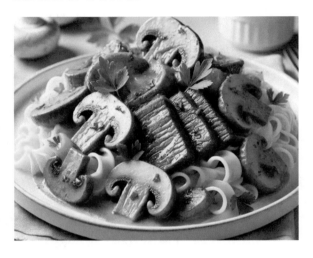

Serves: 1

Cooking Time: 30 minutes

Ingredients and Portions/Measurements:

- Beef Sirloin (Noom diet red coded friendly): 4 ounces, thinly sliced (High in protein, moderate in fat)
- Mushrooms (Noom diet red coded friendly): 1/2 cup, sliced (Low in calories, adds flavor and texture)
- Olive Oil (Minimal amount for cooking): 1 teaspoon (Healthy fat, use sparingly)
- Onion (Noom diet red coded friendly): 1/4 cup, finely chopped (Adds flavor and nutrients)
- Garlic (Noom diet red coded friendly): 1 clove, minced (Adds flavor and has health benefits)
- Beef Broth (Low-sodium, Noom diet red coded friendly): 1/4 cup (Adds flavor and moisture)
- Sour Cream (Noom diet red coded friendly): 2 tablespoons (Adds creaminess and flavor)
- Dijon Mustard (Noom diet red coded friendly): 1 teaspoon (Adds tangy flavor)
- Salt (Noom diet red coded friendly): A pinch (Enhances flavor)
- Black Pepper (Noom diet red coded friendly): To taste (Adds flavor without calories)
- Fresh Parsley (Optional, for garnish): 1 tablespoon, chopped (Adds flavor and nutrients)
- Whole Wheat Egg Noodles (Noom diet red coded friendly): 1/2 cup, cooked (Provides carbohydrates and fiber)

Instructions:

- Heat the olive oil in a non-stick skillet over medium heat.
- Add the finely chopped onion and minced garlic to the skillet. Sauté for about 2-3 minutes until fragrant.

- Add the sliced beef sirloin to the skillet. Cook for about 4-5 minutes until browned and cooked through.
- Remove the beef from the skillet and set aside.
- In the same skillet, add the sliced mushrooms. Cook for about 5 minutes until tender.
- Add the beef broth, sour cream, and Dijon mustard to the skillet. Stir to combine and bring to a simmer.
- Return the cooked beef to the skillet and cook for another 2-3 minutes until heated through.
- Season with salt and black pepper to taste.
- Serve the beef stroganoff over cooked whole wheat egg noodles.
- Garnish with fresh parsley if desired.
- Enjoy your Beef Stroganoff with Mushrooms immediately!

Scientific Note:

Beef sirloin is a high-protein food that provides essential amino acids necessary for muscle repair and growth. However, it is also moderate in fat and should be consumed in moderation as part of a balanced diet. Protein helps maintain muscle mass and supports overall body functions.

Whole wheat egg noodles provide carbohydrates and fiber, which aid in digestion and help maintain a feeling of fullness. While they are considered a red-coded food due to their refined nature, they can be enjoyed in controlled portions as part of a balanced diet.

This recipe aligns with the Noom diet principles by providing a nutrient-dense, moderate-calorie dinner that includes red-coded foods in a controlled portion. It emphasizes balance and moderation, allowing for the enjoyment of all foods within the context of a healthy diet.

Nutritional Information (per serving):

- Calories: ~450
- Protein: 30g
- Total Fat: 20g
- Fiber: 5g
- Sodium: Moderate

BBQ Pork Tenderloin with Sweet Potatoes

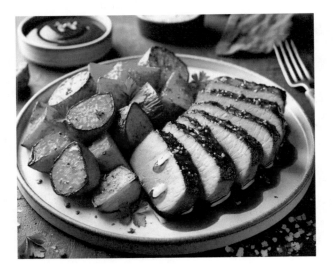

Serves: 1

Cooking Time: 35 minutes

Ingredients and Portions/Measurements:

Pork Tenderloin (Noom diet red coded friendly): 5 ounces (High in protein, moderate in fat)

- BBQ Sauce (Noom diet red coded friendly): 2 tablespoons (Adds flavor)
- Sweet Potato (Noom diet red coded friendly): 1 small, diced (Provides fiber and complex carbohydrates)
- Olive Oil (Minimal amount for cooking): 1 teaspoon (Healthy fat, use sparingly)
- Salt (Noom diet red coded friendly): A pinch (Enhances flavor)
- Black Pepper (Noom diet red coded friendly): To taste (Adds flavor without calories)
- Garlic Powder (Noom diet red coded friendly): 1/2 teaspoon (Adds flavor)
- Fresh Parsley (Optional, for garnish): 1 tablespoon, chopped (Adds flavor and nutrients)

Instructions:

- Preheat the oven to 400°F (200°C).
- Season the pork tenderloin with salt, black pepper, and garlic powder.
- Heat the olive oil in a skillet over medium-high heat.
- Sear the pork tenderloin in the skillet for about 2-3 minutes on each side until browned.
- Transfer the pork tenderloin to a baking dish and brush with BBQ sauce.
- Place the diced sweet potato in the same baking dish around the pork. Season with a pinch of salt and black pepper.
- Bake in the preheated oven for 25-30 minutes, or until the pork reaches an internal temperature of 145°F (63°C) and the sweet potatoes are tender.
- Remove from the oven and let the pork rest for a few minutes before slicing.

- Serve the BBQ pork tenderloin with the roasted sweet potatoes.
- Garnish with fresh parsley if desired.
- Enjoy your BBQ Pork Tenderloin with Sweet Potatoes immediately!

Scientific Note:

Pork tenderloin is a high-protein food that provides essential amino acids necessary for muscle repair and growth. It is also relatively low in fat compared to other cuts of pork, making it a healthier option. Protein helps maintain muscle mass and supports overall body functions.

BBQ sauce adds flavor to the dish, but it can also contain added sugars and sodium. Using it sparingly helps enhance the taste without significantly increasing calorie content.

Nutritional Information (per serving):

- Calories: ~400
- Protein: 30g
- Total Fat: 10g
- Fiber: 4g
- Sodium: Moderate

CHAPTER 5

14 DAYS MEAL PLAN

Day 1:

Breakfast (Green): Spinach and Mushroom Scramble

Lunch (Green): Zesty Citrus and Herb Salad

Dinner (Yellow): Lemon Herb Chicken with Quinoa

Day 2:

Breakfast (Yellow): Banana Almond Overnight Oats

Lunch (Green): Zucchini Noodles with Lemon Herb Dressing

Dinner (Green): Cauliflower Rice Stir-Fry

Day 3:

Breakfast (Green): Watermelon Mint Smoothie

Lunch (Yellow): Mediterranean Quinoa Salad

Dinner (Yellow): Spaghetti Squash with Tomato Basil Sauce

Day 4:

Breakfast (Green): Kale and Apple Breakfast Salad

Lunch (Green): Asian-Inspired Cabbage Wraps

Dinner (Red): Grilled Steak with Garlic Butter

Day 5:

Breakfast (Yellow): Greek Yogurt Parfait with Granola and Berries

Lunch (Green): Tangy Radish and Herb Salad

Dinner (Green): Spinach and Mushroom Stuffed Portobello

Day 6:

Breakfast (Green): Cantaloupe and Berry Breakfast Bowl

Lunch (Yellow): Spicy Chickpea and Avocado Wrap

Dinner (Yellow): Chickpea and Vegetable Stir-Fry

Day 7:

Breakfast (Green): Fresh Garden Veggie Scramble

Lunch (Green): Mango and Cucumber Summer Roll

Dinner (Red): BBQ Pork Tenderloin with Sweet Potatoes

Week 2

Day 8:

Breakfast (Yellow): Sweet Potato and Spinach Breakfast Hash

Lunch (Yellow): Lentil and Vegetable Stuffed Bell Pepper

Dinner (Green): Eggplant and Tomato Bake

Day 9:

Breakfast (Green): Watermelon Mint Smoothie

Lunch (Green): Zucchini Noodles with Lemon Herb Dressing

Dinner (Yellow): Baked Cod with Mango Salsa

Day 10:

Breakfast (Yellow): Apple Cinnamon Oatmeal

Lunch (Green): Tangy Radish and Herb Salad

Dinner (Green): Cabbage and Carrot Stir-Fry

Day 11:

Breakfast (Red): Classic Pancake with Maple Syrup

Lunch (Yellow): Chicken and Avocado Salad Wrap

Dinner (Yellow): Moroccan-Spiced Lentil Stew

Day 12:

Breakfast (Green): Kale and Apple Breakfast Salad

Lunch (Yellow): Tuna and Quinoa Salad

Dinner (Green): Lemon Herb Zoodle Salad

Day 13:

Breakfast (Green): Spinach and Mushroom Scramble

Lunch (Green): Asian-Inspired Cabbage Wraps

Dinner (Red): Beef Stroganoff with Mushrooms

Day 14:

Breakfast (Yellow): Savory Sweet Potato Breakfast Bowl

Lunch (Green): Zesty Citrus and Herb Salad

Dinner (Yellow): Spaghetti Squash with Tomato Basil Sauce

WEEKLY MEAL PLANNER <u>1</u>

MONDAY

BREAKFAST _____

LUNCH _____

SNACKS _____

DINNER _____

TUESDAY

BREAKFAST _____

LUNCH _____

SNACKS _____

DINNER _____

WEDNESDAY

BREAKFAST _____

LUNCH _____

SNACKS _____

DINNER _____

THURSDAY

BREAKFAST _____

LUNCH _____

SNACKS _____

DINNER _____

FRIDAY

BREAKFAST _____

LUNCH _____

SNACKS _____

DINNER _____

SATURDAY

BREAKFAST _____

LUNCH _____

SNACKS _____

DINNER _____

SUNDAY

BREAKFAST _____

LUNCH _____

SNACKS _____

DINNER _____

NOTES

_____

_____

_____

_____

WEEKLY MEAL PLANNER __2__

MONDAY

BREAKFAST _____

LUNCH _____

SNACKS _____

DINNER _____

TUESDAY

BREAKFAST _____

LUNCH _____

SNACKS _____

DINNER _____

WEDNESDAY

BREAKFAST _____

LUNCH _____

SNACKS _____

DINNER _____

THURSDAY

BREAKFAST _____

LUNCH _____

SNACKS _____

DINNER _____

FRIDAY

BREAKFAST _____

LUNCH _____

SNACKS _____

DINNER _____

SATURDAY

BREAKFAST _____

LUNCH _____

SNACKS _____

DINNER _____

SUNDAY

BREAKFAST _____

LUNCH _____

SNACKS _____

DINNER _____

NOTES

_____

_____

_____

_____